W9-BJH-347

PRACTICAL STRESS MANAGEMENT

A Comprehensive Workbook for Managing Change and Promoting Health

SECOND EDITION

John A. Romas
Minnesota State University, Mankato

Manoj Sharma
University of Nebraska at Omaha

ALLYN AND BACON

Boston • London • Toronto • Sydney • Tokyo • Singapore

Vice President, Editor-in-Chief: *Paul A. Smith*
Publisher: *Joseph E. Burns*
Editorial Assistant: *Tanja Eise*
Marketing Manager: *Richard Muhr*
Composition and Prepress Buyer: *Linda Cox*
Manufacturing Buyer: *David Repetto*
Cover Administrator: *Jenny Hart*
Production Administrator: *Deborah Brown*
Editorial-Production Service: *P. M. Gordon Associates*
Text Designer: *Publishers' Design and Production Services, Inc.*

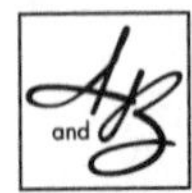

Copyright © 2000, 1995 by Allyn & Bacon
A Pearson Education Company
160 Gould Street
Needham Heights, Massachusetts 02494

Internet: www.abacon.com

All rights reserved. No part of the material protected by this copyright notice may be reproduced or utilized in any form or by any means, electronic or mechanical, including photocopying, recording, or by any information storage and retrieval system, without the written permission of the copyright owner.

Library of Congress Cataloging-in-Publication Data

Romas, John Albert.
Practical stress management : a comprehensive workbook for managing change and promoting health / John A. Romas, Manoj Sharma.
—2nd ed.
p. cm.
Includes bibliographical references and index.
ISBN 0-205-31132-6 (pbk. : alk. paper)
1. Stress management. I. Sharma, Manoj. II. Title.
RA785.R65 2000
155.9′042—dc21 99-35928
CIP

Printed in the United States of America
10 9 8 7 6 5 4 03 02 01 00 99

May our children aspire to become the ones they dream to be
and bring sunshine to themselves as well as others.

To Judi and Jennifer
and
Mom and Dad

J. A. Romas

To Mummy, Daddy, and Guruji
and
Sulekha, Ankita, and Malvika

M. Sharma

Contents

List of Illustrations and Tables

Foreword

When invited to write a foreword to a workbook entitled *Practical Stress Management*, I immediately accepted because of the excitement about how useful a personal workbook on managing stress could be. There was also the conviction that the authors would do a thorough and competent job in carrying out the task. A serious human need would thus be met.

The role of a foreword varies greatly from one book to another, while still others get along well without one. In some it becomes an endorsement of the book and/or its authors; in others it functions as an introduction, an overview, or a preface to the document. This one may well be a little of all of these.

That stress is a pervasive presence in Western culture is more than obvious. The pressure to do one's work faster, thus achieving greater productivity, yet with higher quality is the drumbeat of the production economies of the developed world. These forces have often reached well beyond material production and have invaded every aspect of Western life. Since this "pressure" is far from being the main or only source of stress in our society, it is offered here merely as an example of the pervasiveness of the problem. At the risk of oversimplifying the concept, it may be said that stress can be seen as the product of real or perceived friction between the individual and his or her environment. Stress arises from the disharmony one feels between the self and all the forces that impinge upon that self. The authors present a much more comprehensive definition of stress, but perhaps this will serve for the purposes of a foreword.

The concern that so many individuals have in searching for a way or ways to manage or cope with stress provides all the necessary evidence of the need for a workbook such as this. There is a great deal of literature on stress, but a do-it-yourself handbook for the individual who recognizes his/her problem and wants to try to address it is truly lacking. That the workbook can also serve as a course of study or a syllabus for professionals who wish to do training in stress management is an additional advantage. The fact that "students" in the process, whether seeking self-help or preparing to teach others, take away a comprehensive workbook in the techniques is still another plus.

There are a number of features of the workbook that could be cited for their usefulness or special value, but the worksheets stand out. These guides to self-analysis, situation analysis, and problem delineation are particularly worthy of note. The way they have been selected or devised; the topics, issues, or problems they cover; and the developmental or growth processes they follow are especially commendable.

One could not conclude a statement such as this without mentioning the qualifications of the authors. Professor John A. Romas did advanced graduate study here at the University of Michigan while developing his research skills. His continuing work in health promotion and stress reduction as researcher and scholar are viewed with pride. Dr. Sharma we know only by his work. His role as research scholar, his medical expertise, his work in community health and health promotion, and his background in Eastern philosophies and stress management have prepared him well to contribute to this work.

The authors' background in both Western and Eastern cultures has equipped them well to produce this outstanding guide that draws on the philosophical, social, and research reservoirs of both.

Edwin J. McClendon, M.P.H., Ed.D.
Professor Emeritus, Public Health and Health Education
University of Michigan, Ann Arbor, 1994

Preface

We are extremely encouraged by the success of the first edition of this workbook. The readers found the material to be "user-friendly" and pragmatic. We were told by a number of our readers that they found that the techniques presented in this workbook indeed "worked" for them and that the language of the workbook was clear, simple, and to the point. Readers considered the several worksheets in each of the ten chapters to be a remarkable "strength" of the material. They regarded the workbook's "cafeteria" approach of presenting a multitude of different techniques as a major asset that allowed them to pick and choose the most relevant techniques for their particular situations. In addition to its student readers from academic settings, this workbook has been popular among general readers in various walks of life who have applied the techniques presented herein and benefited from them.

Some of the readers and reviewers of our workbook, however, expressed the need to separate out the major and minor topics, especially for the student readership in colleges and universities. The Eastern concepts posed special challenges, primarily because of the vocabulary. Therefore, in this revised second edition each chapter presents a box that deals with some of the minor topics, which though interesting for the readers, can be excluded, from the point of view of examining the students within the academic setting. They also include some topics that may be considered more recent. The boxes are entitled:

- Ancient Concepts of Stress in the East
- The Health Belief Model and Its Application to Stress Management
- Yoga and Meditation
- Computer Technology Advances: Newer Challenges for Stress Awareness
- Tips on Managing Anger Based on Eastern Philosophy
- Emotional Intelligence
- Caffeine: What It Is and How Much Is Found in Popular Drinks
- Physical Activity: Benefits and Recommendations from the Surgeon General's Report
- Time Waster Personalities
- Eastern Views on Obtaining Results

In this edition we have updated the textual material and references. On demand from our readers, we have also developed an accompanying audio CD on relaxation that includes basic techniques on Yogic Breathing (*Pranayama*), Progressive Muscle Relaxation, Autogenic Training, and Visual Imagery. The audio CD will be a useful aid to the workbook in helping readers to acquire relaxation techniques more easily.

We are thankful to all of the reviewers who read through the first edition of the workbook. A special appreciation is extended to Daniel W. Zenga, Ed.D., L.P., always a friend, who helped us learn to practice what we have written and to understand that in managing stress we are really managing ourselves. In addition, we would like to acknowledge and thank Patricia J. Lussky, M.S., health educator and counselor, for taking the time to prepare our introduction to the audio CD on relaxation. We are indebted to Dr. Kent K. Kalm for his valued time and abilities in preparing the audio CD. We would also like to acknowledge Kristin A. Woizeschke, health resource librarian, Immanuel St. Joseph's–Mayo Health System, Mankato Minnesota, for her expertise in checking through each chapter reference.

J. A. Romas and M. Sharma
Summer 1999

Preface to the First Edition

Health promotion is the process of enabling people to increase control over, and to improve, their health. To reach a state of complete physical, mental, and social well-being, an individual or group must be able to identify and to realize aspirations to satisfy needs, and to change or cope with the environment. Health is, therefore, seen as a resource for everyday life, not the objective of living.

—Ottawa Charter for Health Promotion, 1986
First International Conference on Health Promotion

One of the most remarkable developments of recent years has been the interest shown in health promotion by health professionals all over the world. There is a growing trend in health care of shifting emphasis from curative, institutionalized care to promotive, preventive self-care. It has generally been recognized and accepted that people should exert greater control over their behaviors in order to lead a productive, satisfying, and balanced life. Furthermore, there are numerous rapid advances in technology that have resulted in changes greatly affecting modern life. Inherent in these changes is stress. It is within this context that we address the adverse effects of stress, thereby reducing risk factors that contribute to many stress-related diseases. By managing stress constructively and positively, we can prevent the adverse effects of disease from occurring and enhance our quality of life.

Human beings throughout history have struggled with and managed stress successfully. Paralleling the development of most fields, stress management has become a scientific discipline. The basics of stress management have been derived from the fields of physiology, psychology, medicine, health behavior, health education, and philosophy—particularly Eastern systems like Yoga, Zen, Rinzai, Sufism, and others. But the scientific component aside, stress management is also an art, as each individual is a different entity whose differences need to be dealt with appropriately.

We are presenting to our readers a pragmatic approach to stress management in a simple language. Our emphasis is on practicality based upon scientific research and documented techniques. We have provided a workbook format that is reader-friendly. Worksheets, Thoughts for Reflection, Stress Management Principles, and Summary Points are provided in each chapter. This approach is not just a compilation of techniques but has been practically tested in the field, is backed by scientific evidence, and is complete and holistic. The workbook is a unique blend of thoughts—contemporary and old, Eastern and Western, medical and behavioral, traditional and scientific. It is geared toward changing our routine thought and behavior patterns and replacing those patterns with practical, action-oriented, healthy thinking patterns to manage stress more effectively. We believe that after reading and practicing the methods described in this workbook, the reader will be able to lead a balanced, peaceful, and satisfying life. We are sure that the reader can also introduce this approach to others. Such efforts can trigger a chain reaction that can help society achieve balance, harmony, and peace. In academic settings this workbook will be useful as a text or supplemental text for students in health science, health promotion/health education, preventive medicine, psychology, management, and allied health professions.

We present this workbook to all those who worry. Some worry over yesterday—for what they could not do, the mistakes they committed, and their aches and pains. Others worry over tomorrow—for what they will do, the adversities they will face, and the blunders they will commit. But, certainly, it is no use to worry over yesterday, because it is not with us anymore, never to return again. And tomorrow has not yet come and may hold innumerable possibilities, but only when the sun rises! Anyone can fight the battle of just one day at a time. It is only when we add the burden of yesterdays and tomorrows that contentment and peace of mind elude us. Therefore, we have to acquire knowledge, develop skills, and foster a positive attitude to deal with today better. This workbook is an attempt to help us achieve these goals, thereby effectively managing change and promoting health.

We wish to acknowledge all the people who have been instrumental in helping us to develop this workbook, particularly those, including our students, who have tried, tested, and benefited from the techniques presented during these past years. We are thankful to all our colleagues and reviewers throughout the nation for providing constructive feedback: Barbara A. Brehm Curtis, Smith College; W. Michael Felts, East Carolina University; Allen Pat Kelly, Essex Community College; Frances McGrath-Kovarik, San Jose State University; James F. McKenzie, Ball State University; Glen J. Peterson, Lakewood Community College; Deborah A. Wuest, Ithaca College; and Kathleen J. Zavela, University of Northern Colorado. We are also thankful to Winston W. Benson, Harry Krampf, Harold Slobof, B. L. Sharma, and Sharon Zablotney for their valuable advice at the initiation of this workbook project. At Allyn and Bacon, our publishers, we are grateful to Kevin Stone, Laura Pearson, and Suzy Spivey, editors; Joe Burns, publisher, Health, Physical Education, and Recreation; and Sue Walther Jones, editorial assistant, Health, Physical Education, and Recreation, for their contributions during the various stages of this workbook. We would also like to thank Maria P. Szarke, clinical dietitian at Immanuel St. Joseph's Hospital, Mankato, Minnesota, for providing us with updated information on nutrition, and Krystyna M. Romas for providing excellent editorial comments. Finally, we are much obliged to our families for their sacrifice, continued love, and support.

J. A. Romas and M. Sharma

CHAPTER 1

Understanding Stress

The Human Seasons

Four Seasons fill the measure of the year;
There are four seasons in the mind of man:
He has his lusty Spring, when fancy clear
Takes in all beauty with an easy span:

He has his Summer, when luxuriously
Spring's honey'd cud of youthful thought he loves
To ruminate, and by such dreaming high
Is nearest unto heaven: quiet coves

His soul has in its Autumn, when his wings
He furleth close; contented so to look
On mists in idleness—to let fair things
Pass by unheeded as a threshold brook.

He has his Winter too of pale misfeature,
Or else he would forego his moral nature.

—John Keats

What Is Stress?

If asked whether or not we have experienced stress in our lives, it is quite likely most of us would respond affirmatively. However, if asked to *define stress* we may not be able to find appropriate words to express ourselves. Our responses would include words such as

- Pressure
- Being down
- Anger
- Anxiety
- Nervousness

- Having butterflies in the stomach
- Strain
- Negative stimulation
- Being uptight
- Depressed
- Being under the weather
- Tension
- Being upset

It is certainly true that these terms convey a meaning of stress. However, in order to comprehend stress completely, we need to explore the meaning of stress in depth. Before you proceed any further, review your knowledge, attitudes, and coping skills pertaining to stress with the help of Worksheets 1.1, 1.2, and 1.3.

Worksheet 1.1
What Do You Know about Stress?

We all have some knowledge about stress. However, much of what we know about stress is based on intuition. We have opinions, beliefs, biases, hunches, and misinformation on the basis of which we perceive stress. The following ten questions are designed to provide you with some feedback regarding what you know about stress. Read each statement and mark T (true) or F (false).

____ 1. One major stressful event like a death of someone close is much more important in causing ill effects of stress than small everyday hassles.

____ 2. Stressors will always precipitate stress.

____ 3. Stress decreases the amount of saliva in the mouth resulting in a feeling of cotton mouth.

____ 4. During stress, energy is conserved.

____ 5. People who are not competitive and have no time urgency are not successful in life and have more stress.

____ 6. A person who often says no loses many friends and ends up having stress.

____ 7. Drinking coffee or tea reduces stress.

____ 8. The good thing about smoking is that it relaxes the body and relieves stress.

____ 9. Exercise helps to build the body but robs it of vital energy causing stress.

____ 10. Acquired behaviors for stress cannot be changed.

FEEDBACK ON WORKSHEET 1.1

1. F Research shows that everyday hassles are even more detrimental to one's health than major life changes (Lazarus, 1984; Monroe & McQuaid, 1994).

2. F Stressors only have the *potential* of eliciting stress. The important thing is how we react (Greenberg, 1999; J. C. Smith, 1993).

3. T Stress leads to two basic physiological processes—stimulation of the autonomic nervous system and the endocrine system. One of the manifestations of these physiological effects is dry mouth (Guyton, 1991).

4. F During stress the sympathetic nervous system is activated resulting in expenditure of energy (Greenberg, 1999; Selye, 1936).

5. F Research shows that people characterized by excessive competitive drive, aggressiveness, impatience, and a hurrying sense of time urgency (Type A) are more prone to stress than people with Type B personality traits characterized by no free-floating hostility, no time urgency, and little competitive spirit (Friedman & Rosenman, 1959).

6. F Saying no—expressing oneself and satisfying one's own needs while not hurting others—is assertiveness and helps to reduce stress (Bower & Bower, 1976; Fensterheim & Fensterheim, 1975; M. J. Smith, 1975).

7. F Colas, coffee, tea, and chocolate contain caffeine, which is a pseudostressor or a sympathomimetic drug that results in a stresslike reaction (Girdano, Everly, & Dusek, 1996; Greenberg, 1999).

8. F Nicotine found in tobacco is also a sympathomimetic agent (Greenberg, 1999).

9. F Exercise is good not only for physical health but also for psychological well-being (United States Department of Health and Human Services, 1996).

10. F The basis for stress management programs is that by reducing stressful behaviors and increasing healthful behaviors, one can better manage stress in life (Enelow & Henderson, 1975; Green & Kreuter, 1991; Kasl & Cobb, 1966).

* * * * *

Worksheet 1.2
How Are Your Stress Coping Skills?

We all cope with stress in our lives. However, some of us are overwhelmed by it. Likewise, some situations trigger more stress for us than others. The following ten statements are designed to provide you with some feedback regarding your coping skills with regard to stress. Please read each statement and rate your skill.

Item	*Excellent*	*Very Good*	*Satis-factory*	*Needs Improve-ment*	*Needs a Lot of Improvement*
1. Ability to relax whenever I want to relax					
2. Ability to assert myself while communicating					
3. Ability to keep my anger under control					
4. Ability to resolve conflicts at work and home					
5. Ability to manage time effectively					
6. Ability to exercise regularly					
7. Ability to cope with anxiety over *future* events					
8. Ability to cope with anxiety over *past* events					

Worksheet 1.2 How Are Your Stress Coping Skills? (cont'd)

Item	*Excellent*	*Very Good*	*Satis-factory*	*Needs Improve-ment*	*Needs a Lot of Improvement*
9. Ability to eat a balanced diet					
10. Ability to set and implement realistic goals in order to accomplish desired objectives in life					

FEEDBACK ON WORKSHEET 1.2

This worksheet enhances your own understanding of the various coping skills that you possess with respect to managing stress in your life. The areas in which you do not have adequate skills can be acquired with patience and practice. The chapters in this workbook will enable you to identify skills that you need to develop further.

* * * * *

Worksheet 1.3
What Kind of Attitude Do You Have about Stress?

All of us have some kind of attitude about stress. While some attitudes are helpful in coping with stress, others are not so helpful. The following ten statements are designed to provide you with some feedback regarding your attitudes about stress. Read each of the following statements and rate yourself.

Item	*Strongly Agree*	*Agree*	*Disagree*	*Strongly Disagree*
1. People with stress are weak-minded.				
2. Stress management programs are never successful.				
3. Stress management programs help people.				
4. Stress cannot be managed.				
5. There is nothing like "stress."				
6. Other people cause my stress.				
7. I never experience stress, but other people around me are stressed.				
8. Stress is not harmful.				

Worksheet 1.3 What Kind of Attitude Do You Have about Stress? (cont'd)

Item	*Strongly Agree*	*Agree*	*Disagree*	*Strongly Disagree*
9. The more we worry about future happenings, the better we can shape them.				
10. If one sets a goal, makes a plan, and implements the plan, then his/her stress levels can be reduced.				

FEEDBACK ON WORKSHEET 1.3

1. All of us experience stress from time to time, and it is not a question of being weak-minded or not.

2–4. Evidence exists that stress management programs are successful in reducing the levels of stress that we experience in our lives. These programs substantially reduce stress and the harmful negative consequences associated with stress.

5. Scientific research demonstrates that all of us experience stress from time to time; the only difference is in how we react to it. Denial leads us nowhere. Prudence lies in accepting reality and finding out the most appropriate way for dealing with stress in our lives.

6. No other person can disturb our peace of mind if we choose not to be disturbed. Therefore, no one else except ourselves can be held responsible for our stress.

7. We have to be careful not to project stress. All of us encounter stress in our lives.

8. Stress has been known to be associated (directly and indirectly) with a variety of disorders like hypertension, coronary heart disease, stroke, headaches, and bronchial asthma (Greenberg, 1999). Denying that stress is harmful is a negative attitude that hinders our learning about the basics of stress management in our lives.

9. Worrying about the future only adds to our stress and is of no use.

10. Scientific evidence indicates that setting a goal and implementing a plan to achieve it is an effective way to reduce stress.

* * * * *

Contemporary Concepts of Stress in the West

According to *Webster's New World Dictionary of American English* (1997, 3rd ed.), the word "stress" is derived from the Latin word *strictus,* meaning hardship, adversity, or affliction. It later evolved as *estresse* in Old French and *stresse* in Middle English. It has been used in the physical sciences, medical science, psychology, and behavioral sciences. Stress has been defined from three perspectives, namely environmental or *external* to the body, as a mental or *internal* state of tension, and the body's own *physical* reaction (Rice, 1999). We shall present this concept of stress as it has evolved in the West from response-based to event-based, and then to the interactional model.

I. Response-Based Concept of Stress

In the Western world, the first attempts at defining stress in a psychological and behavioral context originated with the work of physiologist Walter B. Cannon, who defined stress as a "fight or flight" syndrome; that is, when an organism is stressed, it responds either by fighting with the stressor or by running away from it (Cannon, 1932). This concept gained further understanding with the work of Hans Selye on the *General Adaptation Syndrome* (Selye, 1936, 1974a, 1974b, 1982). While attempting to isolate a new sex hormone in rats, he observed that when injected with ovarian extracts, their adrenal glands (endocrine glands located over the kidneys that pour their secretions directly into the bloodstream) secreted corticoid hormones (a steroid), their thymus and lymph nodes became smaller in size, and they developed stomach ulcers. Later, he found that disparate events like cold, heat, infection, injury, loss of blood, and pain also produced similar responses. He labeled this gamut of responses as the General Adaptation Syndrome (GAS), comprising the following three phases (Figure 1.1):

- **Phase 1: Alarm Reaction.** In the alarm-reaction phase the organism's "homeostasis" or balance is disrupted. The endocrine glands become active—particularly the adrenal glands (secreting corticosteroids), which supply a ready source of energy to the body. This is accompanied by a shrinkage of lymphatic structures, decrease in blood volume, and ulcers in the stomach.

- **Phase 2: Stage of Resistance.** The stage of resistance occurs with continued exposure to the agent that elicited the response. In this stage alarm-reaction changes cease and opposite changes occur, such as increase in blood volume. But the adaptation energy continues to get depleted.

- **Phase 3: Exhaustion.** When exhaustion occurs, permanent damage to the system results. If the agent is not removed, depletion of all energy of the organism takes place and death may ensue.

On this basis, Hans Selye defined stress as "a nonspecific response of the body to any demand made upon it" (Selye, 1936, 1974a, 1974b, 1982). Selye, in his later work, found that the same arousal response can be evoked by different situations. Situations that are productive to the organism he labeled as *eustress;* others that are harmful he labeled as *distress* (Selye, 1982). This model of stress was based on response and was physiological in its orientation. The main criticism leveled at this conceptualization has been its neglect of the situational and individual contexts in which stress occurs (Genest & Genest, 1987).

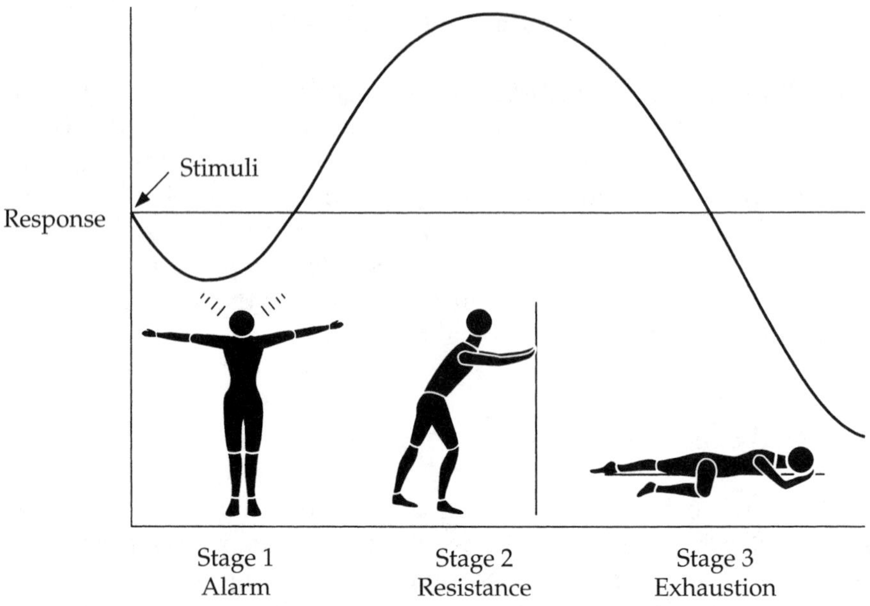

Figure 1.1 Stages of Selye's General Adaptation Syndrome

II. Event-Based Concept of Stress

Thomas Holmes and Richard Rahe (1967) focused on stressful events and constructed a Social Readjustment Rating Scale (SRRS) to assess the amount of stress to which an individual is exposed. The scale developed by Holmes and Rahe (1967) assesses stress by applying weighted life change units to the events in a person's life. These weights are based upon the estimated amount of change or readjustment required for each event on the part of the individual experiencing it. Estimates of this scale have been derived from ratings obtained from a sample of primarily white, middle-class adults. The total life stress experienced during a period of time is assessed by summing the weights, or life change units, of the 43 events represented on the Social Readjustment Rating Scale. Before you proceed any further, complete Worksheet 1.4 keeping in mind the events that you have experienced during the past year.

Thoughts for Reflection 1.1
Murphy's Laws

Reflecting on some of these statements might provide you with some understanding about the beliefs you have that may be producing stress in your life.

- Nothing is as easy as it looks.
- Everything takes longer than you think.
- If anything can go wrong, it will.
- A day without a crisis is a total loss.
- Inside every large problem is a series of small problems struggling to get out.
- The other line always moves faster.
- Whatever hits the fan will not be evenly distributed.
- No matter how long or hard you shop for an item, after you have bought it, it will be on sale somewhere cheaper.
- Any tool dropped while repairing a car will roll underneath to the exact center.
- You will remember that you forgot to take out the trash when the garbage truck is two doors away.
- Friends come and go, but enemies accumulate.
- The light at the end of the tunnel is the headlamp of an oncoming train.
- The chance of the bread falling with the peanut-butter-and-jelly side down is directly proportional to the cost of the carpet.
- The repair man will never have seen a model quite like yours before.
- Beauty is only skin deep, but ugliness goes clear to the bone.

Note: Adapted from *Murphy's laws* popular in common management parlance.

* * * * *

Worksheet 1.4
The Social Readjustment Rating Scale (SRRS)

Focus on the events that you experienced in the past year. For the events experienced, enter the mean value in the score column.

Rank	*Life Event*	*Mean Value*	*Score*
1	Death of spouse/significant other	100	______
2	Divorce	73	______
3	Marital separation	65	______
4	Jail term	63	______
5	Death of a close family member	63	______
6	Personal injury or illness	53	______
7	Marriage/new life partner	50	______
8	Fired at work	47	______
9	Marital reconciliation	45	______
10	Retirement	45	______
11	Change in health of a family member	44	______
12	Pregnancy	40	______
13	Sex difficulties	39	______
14	Gain of a new family member	39	______
15	Business readjustment	39	______
16	Change in financial state	38	______
17	Death of a close friend	37	______
18	Change to a different line of work	36	______
19	Change in number of arguments with spouse/significant other	35	______

Worksheet 1.4 The Social Readjustment Rating Scale (SRRS) (cont'd)

Rank	*Life Event*	*Mean Value*	*Score*
20	Mortgage over $100,000	31	________
21	Foreclosure of mortgage or loan	30	________
22	Change in responsibilities at work (increase or decrease)	29	________
23	Son or daughter leaving home	29	________
24	Trouble with in-laws	29	________
25	Outstanding personal achievement	28	________
26	Spouse/mate beginning or stopping work	26	________
27	Beginning or ending school	26	________
28	Change in living conditions	25	________
29	Revision of personal habits	24	________
30	Trouble with boss/person in authority	23	________
31	Change in work hours or conditions	20	________
32	Change in residence	20	________
33	Change in schools	20	________
34	Change in recreation	19	________
35	Change in church activities	19	________
36	Change in social activities	18	________
37	Mortgage or loan less than $100,000	17	________
38	Change in sleeping habits	16	________

Worksheet 1.4 The Social Readjustment Rating Scale (SRRS) (cont'd)

Rank	*Life Event*	*Mean Value*	*Score*
39	Change in number of family get-togethers	15	________
40	Change in eating habits	15	________
41	Vacation	13	________
42	Christmas	12	________
43	Minor violations of the law	11	________
		TOTAL	________

Note: Adapted from "The social readjustment scale" by T. H. Holmes & R. H. Rahe, *Journal of Psychosomatic Research, 11,* copyright 1967, Elsevier Science Ltd. Reprinted with permission from Elsevier Science Ltd., Oxford, England. Some items from the original scale have been modified to make them more contemporary.

FEEDBACK ON WORKSHEET 1.4

The total score on this SRRS represents the total life change units experienced by the respondent. The scale assesses stress by applying weighted life change units to the events in a person's life. These weights are based upon the estimated amount of change or readjustment required for each event on the part of the individual experiencing it. These estimates have been derived from a sample of primarily white middle-class adults. Therefore, the levels of life change units are subject to modification depending upon social, cultural, and other demographic variables. Furthermore, some of the events, like mortgage, etc., have lost their contemporary significance. But despite these limitations the scale gives a fair idea regarding the stress that you have experienced in the recent past. This view was very popular in the 1970s, and a lot of research substantiated this viewpoint correlating the higher life change unit scores with illness (Holmes & Masuda, 1974; Holmes, 1979; Rahe & Arthur, 1978).

According to this viewpoint, a life change unit score between 150 and 199 showed a 37 percent chance of these stressors leading to sickness in the following year; scores between 200 and 299 a 51 percent chance, and scores over 300 a 79 percent chance (Holmes & Rahe, 1967).

* * * * *

During the 1970s the life events concept was very popular. Holmes (1979) estimated that as many as 1000 publications appeared based on SRRS during the 1970s. Some other scales were also developed based on this concept—for example, the Recent Life Changes Questionnaire (RLCQ) (Rahe, 1974) and the PERI Life Events Scale (Dohrenwend, Krasnoff, Askenasy, & Dohrenwend, 1978). Based upon this concept, stressors have been defined as life events or changes that produce or have the potential to produce changes within the individual, his or her family, and his or her surroundings. However, later work has challenged even this viewpoint. It has been found that stress reactions differ as a function of neurophysiological level of response, qualities of the stressor, and differences among individuals (Genest & Genest, 1987).

III. Interactional Model of Stress

According to the interactional model of stress, which is largely accepted now, the perception of the stressor by the individual is the most important factor. The degree to which anyone is stressed is influenced by a variety of factors. Richard Lazarus (1966, 1984) identified four stages in the process of stress development. The first stage is the *primary appraisal* of the event. In this stage, based upon previous experiences, knowledge about oneself and knowledge about the event by the individual determines whether he or she is in trouble. If the stressor is perceived to be threatening or has caused harm or loss, then the *secondary appraisal* takes place. If, on the other hand, the event is judged to be irrelevant or poses no threat, then stress does not develop any further. The secondary appraisal essentially constitutes how much control one has over the situation. Based upon this understanding, the individual ascertains what means of control are available to him or her. This is the third stage known as *coping.* Finally, *reappraisal* occurs, as to whether the original stressor has been effectively negated or not. These are some of the models prevalent at present that explain the complex phenomenology of stress.

Stressors

An important aspect of enhancing our understanding of stress is understanding more about *stressors.* These are the environmental happenings that have the potential to produce stress. Stressors in a psychosocial context are the demands from the internal or external environment that we perceive as harmful or threatening (Lazarus & Folkman, 1984). These are generally divided into two general classes: discrete, major, stressful *life events* and ongoing, everyday *chronic stressors* (McLean & Link, 1994).

Life Events or Life Change Events

Wheaton (1994, p. 78) describes a life change event as a "discrete, observable, and (it is thought) objectively reportable event that requires some social and/or psychological adjustment on part of the individual." McLean and Link (1994) have further separated life events into recent stressors (typically considered as those experiences occurring within the past year) and remote stressors (which include childhood events such as physical abuse, sexual abuse, and neglect, as well as other events that occurred before the past year). This categorization of stressors is the same as the categorization that we saw in the discussion of the event-based conceptualization of stress in the preceding section.

Chronic Stressors

Recent research has shown that another category of stressors is more important than the discrete life events, because these are more prevalent. We encounter them every day. Since these occur more frequently, they assume greater importance in our lives. These are labeled chronic stressors. Chronic stressors do not necessarily start as distinct events but develop as continuing problematic conditions, have a longer course of duration, and do not end with a self-limiting resolution (Wheaton, 1994). Based on their nature, McLean and Link (1994) have classified chronic stressors into five types.

The first type consists of *persistent life difficulties* that are perceived to be of long duration and are associated with life events. However, the temporal relationships (time sequence) between persistent life difficulties and life events are "often complicated to untangle" (McLean and Link, 1994, p. 24). Examples of these include any event that requires a prolonged period of adjustment, such as a teenage son or daughter leaving home or an accident involving a family member that leaves the person disabled. The second type of chronic stressors is *role strains* that result from strain within specific roles (such as working, being in a relationship, parenting, taking care of a loved one with a serious ailment, being the breadwinner of the family), and fulfilling multiple roles at the same time. The third category is *chronic strains* that occur from the response of one social group to another. Examples of these include the result of overt and covert, intentional and unintentional discriminatory behaviors due to race, ethnicity, class, gender, sexual orientation, or disability. The fourth category of chronic stressors consists of *community-wide strains,* or stressors that operate at an ecological level such as residing in a high-crime area. The fifth category is *daily hassles,* such as waiting too long in a line or being stuck in traffic.

Another Type of Stressors-Nonevents

Besides acute life events and chronic stressors, the research literature also describes nonevents as stressors. Nonevents have been defined as desired or anticipated events that do not occur or as desirable events that do not occur even though their occurrence is normative for people of a certain group (Wheaton, 1994).

Box 1.1 Ancient Concepts of Stress in the East

One of the ancient civilizations in the world is the one that flourished around the Indus valley and later developed into the civilization in South Asia leading to the country known to the world today as India. We shall be focusing on the concepts drawn from Indian culture and tradition to represent the concept of stress in the East.

The four *Vedas*—the *Rig*, the *Sama*, the *Yajur*, and the *Atharva*—containing over a hundred thousand verses of ancient seers and sages, form the basis of the philosophy of the East. They are supported by the *Upanishads*—108 of which have been preserved. Then there are the 18 *Puranas*, including *Srimad Bhagvatam*, the *Brahma Sutras*, which contain Vedic philosophy in the form of aphorisms, *Yogasutras* of Patanjali, *Tantaras* dealing with esoteric aspects of the spiritual quest, *Manusmriti* containing the codes of conduct, and *Bhagvad Gita*, the gist of *Vedas* (Singh, 1983). In addition, the *Charaka Samhita* and *Susruta Samhita* are the texts of the *Ayurvedic* (Indian) system of medicine.

Stress is depicted by use of terms like *dukha* (meaning pain, misery, or suffering), *klesa* (afflictions), *kama* or *trisna* (desires), *atman* and *ahankara* (self and ego), *adhi* (mental aberrations), and *prajanparadha* (failure or lapse of consciousness) (Pestonjee, 1992). These varied depictions indicate the holistic dimension of stress in Eastern thought. Pestonjee (1992) notes that according to the *Samkhya-yoga* system the cause of stress is *avidya* or faulty reality testing of either or all of the following:

- *Asmita* (self-appraisal)
- *Raga* (object appraisal)
- *Dvesha* (threat appraisal)
- *Abhnivesha* (coping orientation)

According to the Eastern viewpoint, life situations leading to stress can be one of three kinds:

1. *Adhyatmik* (personal), consisting of pathological diseases or psychological afflictions like jealousy, fear, anger, lust, hatred, greed, grandiosity, and depression
2. *Adhibhotik* (situational), consisting of conflicts, competition, aggression, acts of war, and so on
3. *Adhidevik* (environmental), due to natural calamities like earthquake, extremes of temperature, eruption of volcanoes, and so on

Box 1.1 Ancient Concepts of Stress in the East (cont'd)

Stress operates through four levels of stressors:

1. *Prosupta* (Dormant stressors): Any mental process is potentially stressful and can become stressful just as any seed has the potential to germinate into a plant. For example, a student might imagine that he or she is going to be severely reprimanded if he or she is late for class. This imagination would be a dormant stressor.

2. *Tonu* (Tenuous or weak stressors): These are stressors of insufficient intensity and urgency that are kept in check by more powerful stressors. For example, when one is hungry, the hunger response (powerful stressor) would override worrying about being late for class (tenuous or weak stressor).

3. *Vichchinna* (Intercepted stressors): These stressors alternate between stages of dormancy and manifestation. For example, a student who is reprimanded for coming late to class subsequently tries to come on time. The student has a stressor that will manifest when he or she becomes late. This is an intercepted stressor.

4. *Udara* (Operative stressors): These stressors have found complete expression in behavior. For example, a student who has conditioned his or her behavior to be present before time for class is exhibiting this behavior because of an operative stressor.

Hence, Eastern thought primarily places emphasis on the powers of the individual in coping with stress. The individual can, with the help of *vidya* or *gyana* (knowledge and correct perception), understand the situation correctly, with adequate practice (*sadhana*) apply appropriate skills to reduce undue response to stressors and ultimately develop a wholesome attitude devoid of manifest stress (*samadhi bhavana*). This, in simple terms, is an explanation of the Eastern concept of stress that places an emphasis on the "correct perception" of any event by an individual in dealing with stress.

* * * * *

Effects of Stress on the Body

Another aspect of understanding the concept of stress is the effect that stress has on the body. Visualizing these abstract concepts in the form of models is generally a helpful approach to enhance our understanding. Figure 1.2 attempts to present these concepts in a model that is generally well accepted.

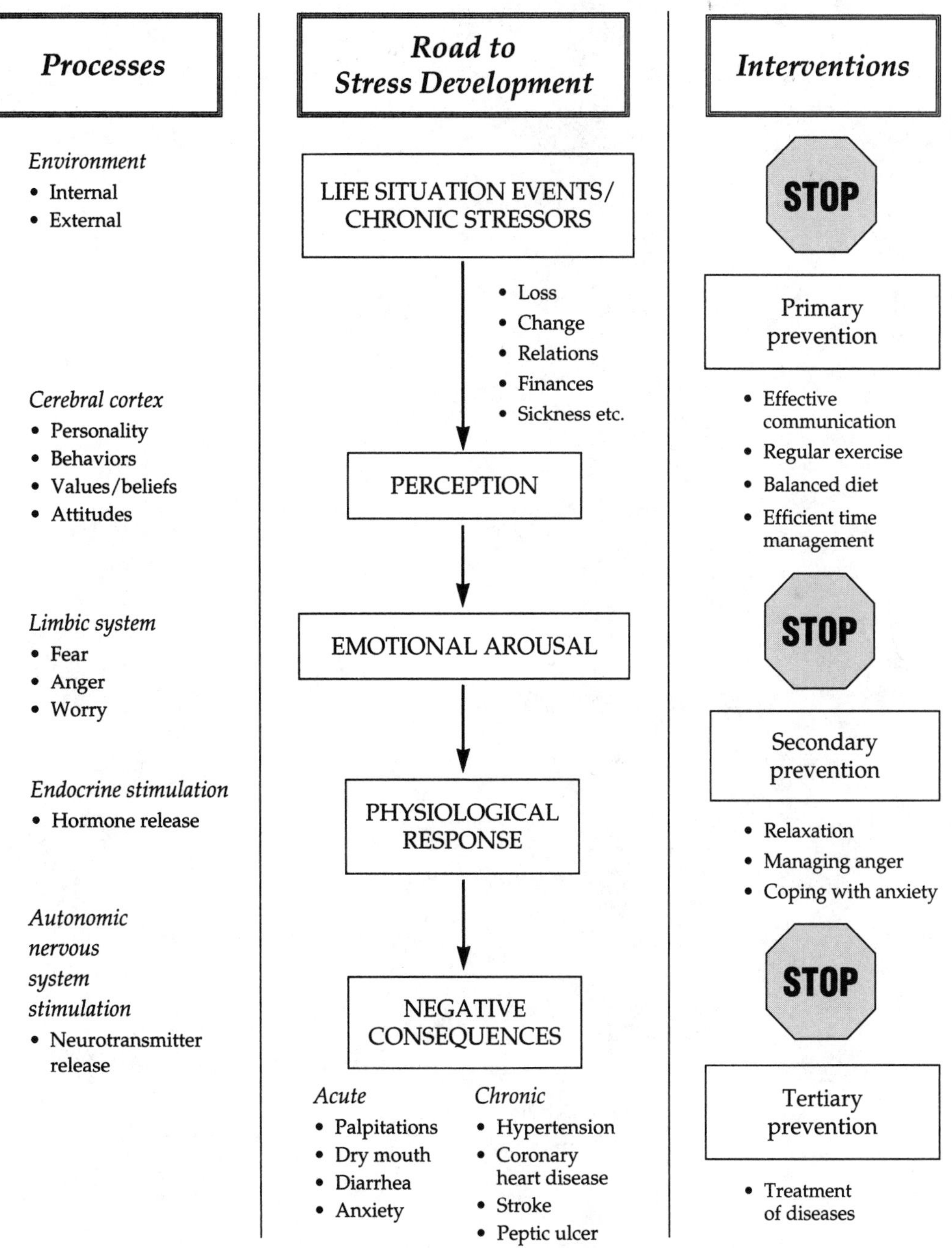

Figure 1.2 Stress: Development and Intervention

Various *life situations* from the internal or external environment, like loss, change, sickness, acute life events, and chronic stressors, might contribute to problematic relationships and poor financial management, which affect us. These stressors are *perceived* by the cerebral cortex, that is the part of the brain which is responsible for judgment, decision making, and other higher functions. This interpretation is modified based upon our personalities, behavioral styles, values, beliefs, norms, and attitudes. Before we proceed any further, identify your personality type with the help of Worksheet 1.5.

Worksheet 1.5
Personality Type Identification

Answer the following questions as either yes or no and count the number of yes responses when completed.

1. Do I accentuate key words in speech and hurry the last few words in my sentences?
2. Do I always eat, walk, talk, and move rapidly?
3. Do I get impatient and irritated when things do not move fast?
4. Do I often attempt to do or think more than one thing at a time?
5. Do I always try to move the topic of conversation to my interest?
6. Do I have feelings of guilt when I relax?
7. Do I frequently fail to take note of new things around me?
8. Am I more concerned with getting things worth having than with becoming what is worth being?
9. Do I suffer from a chronic sense of time urgency?
10. Do I compete or feel compelled to challenge others?
11. Do I engage in expressive gestures like pounding the table, etc., in conversation?
12. Do I believe my fast pace is necessary?
13. Do I rate life's success in terms of "numbers"?

Note: Adapted from *Type A behavior and your heart* (pp. 100–102) by Meyer Friedman and Ray Rosenman, 1974, New York: Fawcett Crest. Copyright © 1974 by Meyer Friedman. Adapted by permission from Alfred A. Knopf, Inc.

FEEDBACK ON WORKSHEET 1.5

If the total number of your yes responses is more than 7, then you are likely to be Type A in your orientation. The higher your score is from 7 toward 13, the stronger is the likelihood of your being Type A. Type A personality types exhibit excessive competitive drive, are aggressive and impatient, and always have an urgency of time. The basis of this personality is believed to be a free-floating form of generalized hostility and a sense of insecurity. If, on the contrary, you have lower scores, you are likely to be Type B in your orientation. Type B personality types do not have an urgency of time, are not competitive; rather they tend to be cooperative and patient. These are the happy-go-lucky kind of people.

Type A personality types have been shown to be more prone to stress and its negative consequences. However, these personality type classifications are not rigid assessments and are more *situational* in their connotation. Importantly, they can be modified.

* * * * *

The way we behave day to day constitutes our behavioral style. This topic is discussed in greater detail in Chapter 4. After perception the next stage in the development of stress is the *emotional response* that triggers activity in the limbic system. The limbic system is the primitive part of the brain that is the seat of various emotions like anger, fear, insecurity, worry, and so on. The emotional arousal activates the *physiological response,* which is manifested in the form of stimulation of the endocrine glands and the autonomic nervous system. The *endocrine glands* are the glands that pour their secretions directly into the bloodstream. These secretions are called hormones. Hormones are essential chemicals that have a wide range of effects on the body. They need to be produced in optimum amounts in order for the body to function normally. An excess or lack of these vital substances can lead to a variety of pathological disorders. The *autonomic nervous system* is that part of the central nervous system (brain and spinal cord) that regulates the functioning of vital organs. It consists of the sympathetic and the parasympathetic nervous system. In simplistic terms it can be said that the sympathetic nervous system is the one that is responsible for spending energy, and the parasympathetic nervous system is the one responsible for conserving energy in the body. Figure 1.3 depicts the complex physiological changes that take place in the body as a result of stress.

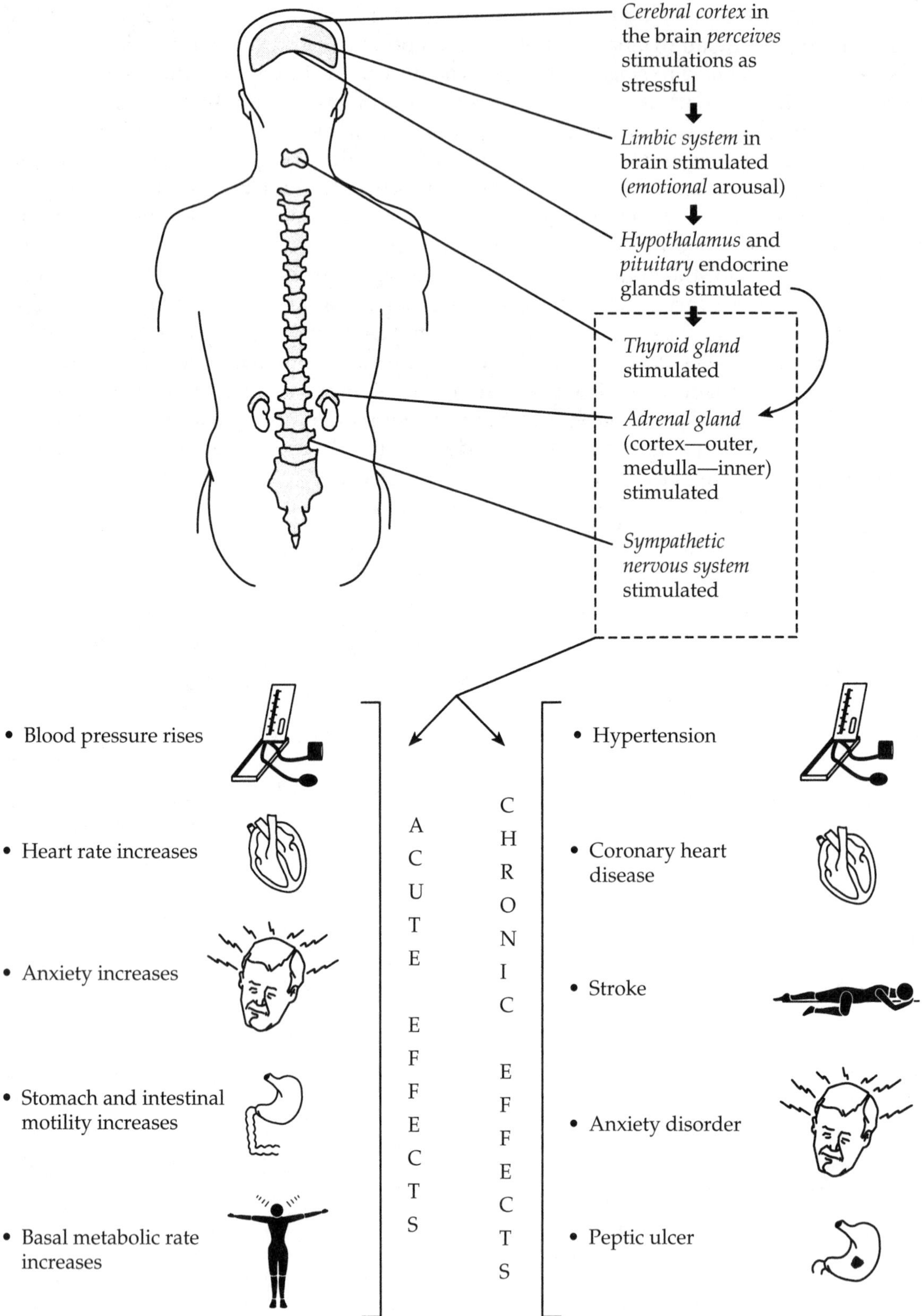

Figure 1.3 Stress Psychophysiology

The net result of both these physiological activities (endocrine and autonomic nervous system stimulation) is that a variety of chemicals are produced in the body. More often than not these chemical by-products do not get used and accumulate within the body. These chemical by-products are responsible for the *negative consequences* in the body. Stress produces both acute or short-term immediate effects and chronic or long-term effects. Figure 1.4 presents the various immediate signs and symptoms of acute stress on the human body.

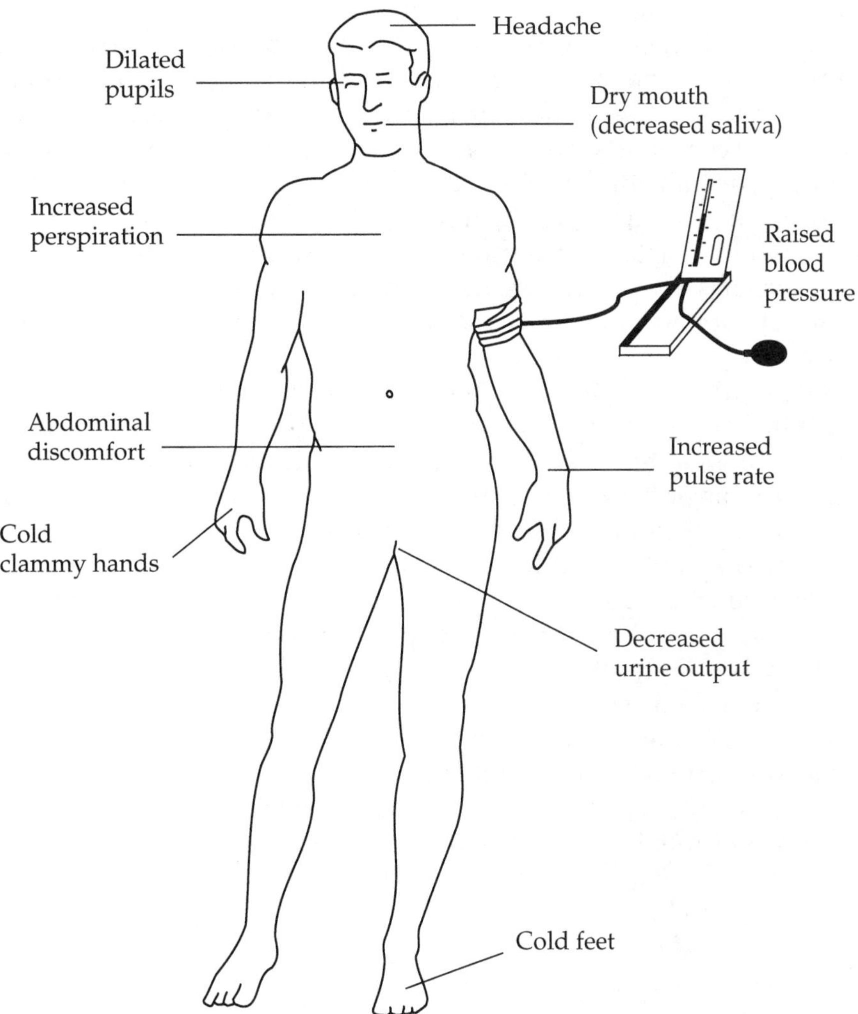

Figure 1.4 Physiological Signs and Symptoms of Acute Stress on the Body

Stress, because of its chronic effects, can be a direct causative factor, an indirect contributory factor, a precipitating factor, or an aggravating factor for various diseases. Some of the pathological signs, symptoms, and diseases commonly associated with stress are anxiety disorders, insomnia, hypertension, stroke, coronary heart disease, ulcers, migraine headaches, tension headaches, rheumatoid arthritis, temporomandibular joint syndrome, bronchial asthma, and backache (Greenberg, 1999; Rice, 1999).

Stress in the Overall Context

Until now, we have discussed the concept of stress from an Eastern and Western perspective, how it has developed over time, and what the effects of stress are on the human body. This discussion has been medical, physiological, philosophical, and behavioral in its connotation. What is also required in this conceptualization is the historical, sociocultural, political, and organizational context in which we experience stress.

From time immemorial, human life has always been ridden with stress. In premodern times there were greater threats from natural calamities, extremes of temperature, pestilence, and so on. In modern times, while industrialization has provided many facilities and improvement in the physical quality of life for many of us, these stressors have been replaced by a faster pace of life, rapidly changing technology, divergence in morality, increasing social complexity, and so on. The student of today, the worker of today, the executive of today, and all other people today, have to face greater stress than their counterparts of yesteryear. Woolfolk and Lehrer (1993) note that present society has become individualistic and materialistic in contrast to the communal and spiritual society of the past. Never before has a large percentage of the population been without durable and dependable social support in its proper and adequate form. This lack indeed is a great source of stress.

In the organizational context, which could be work setting, school setting, and/or community setting, stress has been studied quite extensively. Beer and Newman (1978) have defined job stress in terms of interaction of the person with job-related factors that disrupt or enhance his or her psychological and physiological condition. This organizational stress is further heightened for people in certain specific situations, such as for women who have to accomplish multiple roles and students who are constantly in a phase of transition. In addition, the crisis of the modern human also lies in finding meaning to his or her activities. Often we are unable to attribute meaning and importance to what we are doing in daily life. In the absence of these meaningful activities with coherence and lawfulness, the stress manifestations increase (Antonovsky, 1987; Shepperd and Kashani, 1991). Furthermore, despite all advancements, for a vast majority of people, primarily in the third world, basic stress is still tied into making two ends meet and mustering enough for food, clothing, and shelter. Therefore, understanding historical, sociocultural, political, and organizational factors in our lives is also essential for dealing with and managing stress more effectively. Thoughts for Reflection 1.2 will help you reflect upon some of the factors affecting modern life.

Thoughts for Reflection 1.2
Why Stress Exists

Present-day life is more complex than ever before. A reflection on some of the factors responsible for this complexity will help you cope with stress better. Following is a list of some of these factors:

- *Intricacy of Social Fabric:* In personal and work life we have come to a point where our relationships have become extremely complex and challenging. Much of our life revolves around getting into, being in, and getting out of relationships. All these events are potentially stressful.
- *Divergence in Morality and Ethics:* We have developed a value system that presents us with highly divergent and conflicting standpoints on various aspects of life issues. Adjustments and responses to these contradictions are stressful.
- *Conflicting Expectations:* Most of the time in our work life as well as our personal life we do not know what is being expected of us. This unclarity about our role is a stressful factor.
- *Marginal Communication:* Poor and ineffective communication in our day-to-day life is a major source of discomfort and stress in our lives.
- *Rapid Change in Technology:* The advancement in science and technology has pervaded all walks of life. Inherent in this change is stress.
- *Lack of Proper Training to Do What One Is Being Asked to Do:* Usually in our work life, owing to the gap between "education" and "profession," we are at times unable to do what is being asked of us. This gap is a strong source of stress.
- *Ineffective Management Systems:* Despite the innovation and implementation of a wide variety of management systems that have enhanced production and have been responsible for quality products, we have been unable to develop a management system that completely rids us of stress.
- *Lack of Job Security:* In present times, we do not know if we shall be able to remain in our job or not. This insecurity provides ample stress in life.
- *Limited or No Organizational Loyalty:* These days many of us cannot associate ourselves with the job that we perform and the organization with which we work. This is an extremely stressful factor.
- *Economic Overextension:* Pressure that money exerts in all walks of life is a potent stressor.

* * * * *

A comprehensive stress management program needs to address all these contexts and perspectives in order for the program to be successful. It shall be our attempt in this workbook to try to do justice in this regard.

Another point that needs to be emphasized is that stress management is essentially a preventive approach. In preventive medicine, prevention occurs at three levels: primary, secondary, and tertiary. *Primary prevention* is the level where the intervention occurs before the disease. In stress management it is the level at the stage of "perception" of the stressor. *Secondary prevention* is the level of intervention when the disease process has started. In the case of stress management, it is the stage when emotional arousal and physiological activation have occurred. *Tertiary prevention* is the level when disease has already caused damage. In the case of stress management, it is the stage when negative consequences have already set in and then we intervene. It is akin to stamping out the fire after the inferno has engulfed the property. In this context it is worth noting that some experts view stress as a risk factor; therefore, stress management, according to them, is primary prevention. However, we would like to view stress as a disease in its developmental form and have, therefore, classified stress management with various levels of prevention described previously.

Finally, the importance of one's *perception and attitude* in comprehending stress and dealing with it cannot be overemphasized. Thoughts for Reflection 1.3 reinforces our belief in the importance of developing a *positive attitude,* which is at the core of all stress management efforts. Stress Management Principle 1, at the end of this chapter, is also in line with this ideology. It is hoped that the reader will not only memorize this principle, but also try to incorporate it in his or her life.

Thoughts for Reflection 1.3
On Attitude

- Attitude determines our behavior.
- It is up to each one of us to choose how we react to any situation.
- What happens to you in life has relatively little effect compared to how you react. If you choose to get upset, worked up, and worried, even a small, trivial event, colored with your imagination, may appear to be devastating. However, if you choose to envision the situation in perspective, and not get upset or worried, then your coping skills are enhanced.
- Effort and directed determination are required for changing attitude.
- Understanding the importance of attitude and its impact upon behavior is more significant than being factual, scientific, and analytical.

* * * * *

Stress Management Principle 1

It is not the stressor but your perception of the stress that is important.

Summary Points

- Walter Cannon defined stress as a "fight or flight" syndrome; that is, when an organism is stressed either it responds by fighting with the stressor or running away from it.
- Hans Selye described the *General Adaptation Syndrome* consisting of *Alarm Reaction, Stage of Resistance,* and *Exhaustion.* On this basis he defined stress as the "nonspecific response of the body to any demand made upon it."
- Thomas Holmes and Richard Rahe constructed the Social Readjustment Rating Scale (SRRS) to assess the amount of stress experienced by an individual as a result of changing life events.
- Richard Lazarus described stress development in *four stages*—namely, *Primary Appraisal, Secondary Appraisal, Coping,* and *Reappraisal.*
- Stressors are of two types: (1) acute life events and (2) chronic stressors.
- Acute life events are of two types: (1) recent (within one year) and (2) remote (beyond one year).
- Chronic stressors are of five types: (1) persistent life difficulties, (2) role strains, (3) chronic stressors, (4) community-wide strains, and (5) daily hassles.
- Nonevents have also been defined as stressful because of perceived expectations.
- According to Eastern thought stress is described as *dukha* (pain, misery, suffering), *klesa* (afflictions), *kama* or *trisna* (desires), *atman* and *ahankara* (self and ego), *adhi* (mental aberrations), and *prajanparadha* (failure or lapse of consciousness). The main cause is *avidya* (faulty reality testing).
- Type A personality people (characterized by hurrying nature, competitive zeal, dominating nature, and fast pace of life) are more prone to stress.
- A generally accepted model of stress development consists of life situations that are perceived as stressful and that lead to an emotional and physiological response, thus leading to negative consequences.
- The physiological response in stress basically is composed of endocrine stimulation and sympathetic nervous system overactivity.

- Some pathological signs, symptoms, and diseases associated with stress are anxiety disorders, insomnia, hypertension, stroke, coronary heart disease, ulcers, migraine headaches, tension headaches, rheumatoid arthritis, temporomandibular joint syndrome, bronchial asthma, and backache.
- Stress, besides medical, psychological, behavioral, and philosophical contexts, also needs to be understood in sociocultural, political, and organizational perspectives in order to devise a meaningful stress management effort.

References and Further Readings

Antonovsky, A. (1987). The salutogenic perspective: Toward a new view of health and illness. *Advances, 4,* 47–55.

Beer, T. A., & Newman, H. E. (1978). Job stress, employee health, and organizational effectiveness: A facet analysis, model, and literature review. *Personnel Psychology, 31,* 665–699.

Bower, S. A., & Bower, G. H. (1976). *Asserting your self.* Reading, MA: Addison–Wesley.

Cannon, W. B. (1932). *The wisdom of the body.* New York: W. W. Norton.

Dohrenwend, B. S., Krasnoff, L., Askenasy, A R., & Dohrenwend, B. P. (1978). Exemplification of a method for scaling life events: The PERI Life Events Scale. *Journal of Health and Social Behavior, 19,* 205–229.

Enelow, A. J., & Henderson, J. B. (Eds.). (1975). *Applying behavioral science to cardiovascular risk.* New York: American Heart Association.

Fensterheim, H., & Fensterheim, B. (1975). *Don't say yes when you want to say no.* New York: David McKay.

Friedman, M., & Rosenman, R. H. (1959). Association of specific overt behavior pattern with blood and cardiovascular findings: Blood clotting time, incidence of arcus senilis, and clinical coronary artery disease. *Journal of the American Medical Association, 169,* 1286–1296.

Friedman, M., & Rosenman, R. H. (1974). *Type A behavior and your heart.* New York: Fawcett Crest.

Genest, M., & Genest, S. (1987). *Psychology and health.* Champaign, IL: Research Press.

Girdano, D. A., Everly, G. S., Jr., & Dusek, D. E. (1996). *Controlling stress and tension: A holistic approach* (5th ed.). Englewood Cliffs, NJ: Prentice Hall.

Green, L. W., & Kreuter, M. W. (1991). *Health promotion planning: An educational and environmental approach* (2nd ed.). Mountain View, CA: Mayfield.

Greenberg, J. S. (1999). *Comprehensive stress management* (6th ed.). Boston: William C. Brown/McGraw-Hill.

Guyton, A. C. (1991). *Textbook of medical physiology* (8th ed.). Philadelphia: W. B. Saunders.

Holmes, T. H. (1979). Development and application of a quantitative measure of life change magnitude. In J. E. Barrett, R. M. Rose, & G. L. Klerman (Eds.), *Stress and mental disorder* (pp. 37–53). New York: Raven.

Holmes, T. H., & Masuda, M. (1974). Life change and illness susceptibility. In B. S. Dohrenwend & B. P. Dohrenwend (Eds.), *Stressful life events: Their nature and effects* (pp. 49–72). New York: Wiley.

Holmes, T. H., & Rahe, R. H. (1967). The social readjustment rating scale. *Journal of Psychosomatic Research, 11,* 213–218.

Kasl, S. V., & Cobb, S. (1966). Health behavior, illness behavior, and sick role behavior. *Archives of Environmental Health, 12,* 246–266.

Lazarus, R. S. (1966). *Psychological stress and the coping process.* New York: McGraw-Hill.

Lazarus, R. S. (1984). Puzzles in the study of daily hassles. *Journal of Behavioral Medicine, 7,* 375–389.

Lazarus, R. S., & Folkman, S. (1984). *Stress, appraisal, and coping.* New York: Springer.

McLean, D. E., & Link, B. G. (1994). Unraveling complexity: Strategies to refine concepts, measures, and research designs in the study of life events and mental health. In W. R. Avison & I. H. Gotlib (Eds.), *Stress and mental health: Contemporary issues and prospects for the future* (pp. 15–42). New York: Plenum Press.

Monroe, S. M., & McQuaid, J. R. (1994). Measuring life stress and assessing its impact on mental health. In W. R. Arison & I. H. Gotlib (Eds.), *Stress and mental health: Contemporary issues and prospects for the future* (pp. 43–76). New York: Plenum Press.

Pestonjee, D. M. (1992). *Stress and coping: The Indian experience.* Newbury Park, CA: Sage Publications.

Rahe, R. H. (1974). The pathway between subjects' recent life changes and their near future illness reports: Representative results and methodological issues. In B. S. Dohrenwend & B. P. Dohrenwend (Eds.), *Stressful life events: Their nature and effects* (pp. 73–86). New York: Wiley.

Rahe, R. H., & Arthur, R. J. (1978). Life change and illness studies: Past history and future directions. *Journal of Human Stress, 4,* 3–15.

Rice, P. L. (1999). *Stress and health* (2nd ed.). Pacific Grove, CA: Brooks/Cole.

Selye, H. (1936). A syndrome produced by diverse nocuous agents, *Nature, 138,* 32.

Selye, H. (1974a). *Stress without distress.* Philadelphia: Lippincott.

Selye, H. (1974b). *The stress of life.* New York: McGraw-Hill.

Selye, H. (1982). History and present status of stress concept. In L. Goldberger & S. Breznitz (Eds.), *Handbook of stress: Theoretical and clinical aspects* (pp. 7–17). New York: Free Press.

Sheppard, J. A., & Kashani, J. V. (1991). The relationship of hardiness, gender, and stress to health outcomes in adolescents. *Journal of Personality, 59,* 747–768.

Singh, K. (1983). Hinduism. In *Religions of India* (pp. 17–74). New Delhi, India: Clarion Books.

Smith, J. C. (1993). *Understanding stress and coping.* New York: Macmillan.

Smith, M. J. (1975). *When I say no, I feel guilty.* New York: Dial Press.

United States Department of Health and Human Services. (1996). *Physical activity and health: A report of the Surgeon General* (p. 4). Atlanta: U.S. Department of Health and Human Services, Centers for Disease Control and Prevention, National Center for Chronic Disease Prevention and Health Promotion.

Wheaton, B. (1994). Sampling the stress universe. In W. R. Avison & I. H. Gotlib (Ed.), *Stress and mental health: Contemporary issues and prospects for the future.* New York: Plenum Press.

Woolfolk, R. L., & Lehrer, P. M. (1993). The context of stress management. In P. M. Lehrer & R. L. Woolfolk (Eds.), *Principles and practice of stress management* (2nd ed.) (pp. 3–14). New York: Guilford Press.

CHAPTER 2

Enhancing Awareness about Managing Stress

Infant Innocence

Reader, behold! this monster wild
Has gobbled up the infant child.
The infant child is not aware
It has been eaten by the bear.

—*A. E. Housman*

Awareness about Managing Stress

In the previous chapter we focused on developing knowledge about stress. While knowledge is essential for any behavior change to take place, often it is not sufficient (Bandura, 1995). Besides knowledge, what is also required for behavior change to take place are enhanced personal awareness, appropriate attitudes, suitable beliefs, a well-developed set of skills, and germane environmental conditions (Green & Kreuter, 1991). Since the 1950s behavioral and social scientists have developed several theories and models to enhance our understanding of the complex process of behavioral change (Glanz, Lewis, & Rimer, 1997). One such model is the Health Belief Model, which attempts to explain and predict health behaviors in terms of certain belief patterns (Hochbaum, 1958; Becker, 1974). Box 2.1 presents this model and discusses some beliefs that you need to be aware of in order to manage and reduce stress in your personal life.

It is evident from this model that an understanding of what needs to be changed is an essential starting point for any behavioral change endeavor. Therefore, an understanding of the potential stressors in our life (*cues to action*), potential negative consequences from these stressors (*perceived susceptibility*), and the seriousness of these negative consequences (*perceived severity*) is important for us to begin managing and reducing stress in our personal lives. Therefore, in this chapter we will identify the acute and chronic manifestations of stress in our life, discern some potential personal stressors, and recognize behaviors that need to be changed. In the subsequent chapters of this workbook we will build our confidence in practicing new behaviors that help us manage or reduce stress better in our lives (*self-efficacy*), recognize the benefits of these behaviors (*perceived benefits*), and identify barriers (*perceived barriers*) that prevent us from applying these new behaviors.

Acute Manifestations of Stress

We have already seen in Chapter 1 that stress produces a number of immediate manifestations. These occur soon after a stressor has affected our body. We need to find out what these changes are in our body. Therefore, you should now complete Worksheet 2.1 and find out how your body reacts to acute stress.

Box 2.1 The Health Belief Model and Its Application to Stress Management

The Health Belief Model has several components that attempt to explain or predict behavior change. The following table presents the components of the Health Belief Model and discusses some beliefs that we need to be aware of in order to manage and reduce stress in our personal lives:

Component	*What It Means*	*Stress Managing/ Reducing Beliefs*
Perceived susceptibility	Belief that a person may acquire a disease or enter a harmful state as a result of a particular behavior	If we believe that stress has the potential to produce some *negative consequences* for us, then it is likely that we will act to reduce stress in our lives.
Perceived severity	Belief in the extent of harm that can result from the acquired disease or harmful state as a result of a particular behavior	If we believe that stress has the potential to produce *serious* negative consequences, such as heart disease, then it is likely that we will act to reduce stress in our lives.
Perceived benefits	Belief in the benefit of the methods suggested for reducing the risk or seriousness of the disease or harmful state resulting from a particular behavior	If we believe that by learning stress management techniques, such as relaxation, we will *benefit*, then it is likely that we will follow these new behaviors.
Perceived barriers	Belief concerning actual and imagined costs of following the new behavior	If we can reassure ourselves that applying stress management techniques results in a minimal *expense* and maximal benefit in the long run, then it is likely that we will follow these new behaviors.
Cues to action	Precipitating force that makes a person feel the need to take action	If we can identify the personal stressors that *trigger* negative consequences for us, then it is likely that we will follow the new behaviors that reduce stress in our lives.

Box 2.1 The Health Belief Model and Its Application to Stress Management (cont'd)

Component	*What It Means*	*Stress Managing/ Reducing Beliefs*
Self-efficacy	Confidence to follow a behavior	If we can *practice,* in small steps, new stress management behaviors that we learn in this workbook and demonstrate that we have acquired mastery over these new behaviors, then it is likely that we will follow these new behaviors.

* * * * *

Worksheet 2.1
How Your Body Reacts to Acute Stress

Imagine yourself in a stressful situation. When you are feeling anxious or stressed, what do you typically experience? Check all the items that apply:

____ 1. My heart starts to beat faster and pound harder.

____ 2. I cannot prevent disturbing thoughts from entering my mind.

____ 3. My hands become cold and clammy.

____ 4. I keep brooding on trivial thoughts over and over again.

____ 5. I begin to sweat profusely.

____ 6. I lose the power to concentrate and function effectively.

____ 7. I develop irritable bowel or diarrhea.

____ 8. I cannot make decisions and feel horrible.

____ 9. I cannot sit still and nervously pace up and down.

____ 10. I imagine the worst possible scenario and cannot stop thinking about it.

____ 11. My abdomen begins to hurt.

____ 12. I feel the world around me is crashing and I have lost all control.

____ 13. I feel restless.

____ 14. I imagine horrifying scenes that keep me disturbed for a long time.

____ 15. My body gets stiff, and I am immobilized.

____ 16. I think of leaving everything and just running away.

____ 17. I have a feeling of "butterflies" in my stomach.

____ 18. I want the situation to end favorably as soon as possible but am not sure.

____ 19. I feel tired and exhausted after some time.

____ 20. I develop a headache.

FEEDBACK ON WORKSHEET 2.1

Count the even-numbered and odd-numbered responses separately.

- Odd-numbered responses = ______
- Even-numbered responses = ______

If you have scored more even-numbered responses than odd, then you tend to respond to stress with your *mind.* This result also signifies that you are likely to derive greater relaxation by indulging in the activities of mind like meditation, any interesting hobby, and so on. If you have scored more odd-numbered responses, then your *body* tends to respond more to stress. People who respond to stress by having symptoms in the body generally require systematic physical activity like aerobic exercise, progressive muscle relaxation, and other such techniques. If you have a near equal mixture of even- and odd-numbered responses, then you respond to stress in a *mixed* fashion. A combination of mind relaxation and physical activities is likely to benefit us in relieving our stress.

Note: Based upon personal discussions with Peter R. Kovacek, Henry Ford Hospital, Detroit, MI, 1981.

* * * * *

Chronic Manifestations of Stress

Chronic stress is also harmful to us. Chronic stress can permanently raise our blood pressure levels. This condition is known as hypertension. Hypertension has been identified as a risk factor for coronary heart disease (CHD) and cerebrovascular disease, or stroke. The cause for 90 percent of these cases of hypertension is not known, and these are labeled as essential hypertension (Labarthe & Roccella, 1993). Figure 2.1 shows how stress is related to hypertension and coronary heart disease.

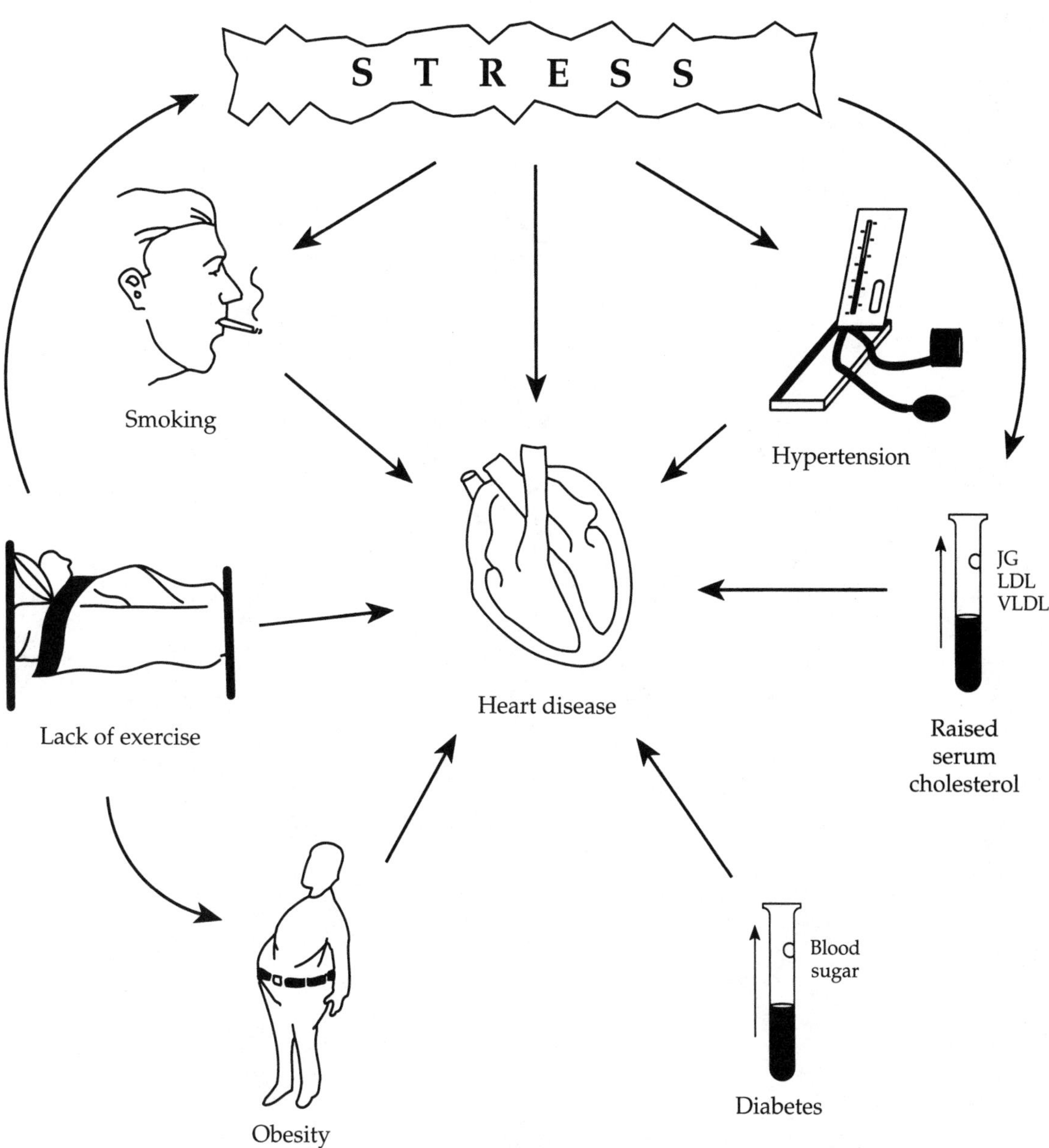

Figure 2.1 Relationship between Stress and Heart Disease

Besides hypertension, coronary heart disease, and stroke, stress is also related as a risk factor to many other physical ailments. Some of these are migraine headaches, peptic ulcers, arthritis, colitis, diarrhea, asthma, cardiac arrhythmias, sexual problems, circulatory problems (cold hands and feet), muscle tension, allergies, backache, temporomandibular joint syndrome, and cancer (Greenberg, 1999; Girdano, Everly, & Dusek, 1997; Rice, 1999; Smith, 1993). Now with the help of Worksheet 2.2, find out whether we experience any manifestations of chronic stress.

Worksheet 2.3, which follows Worksheet 2.2, has been designed to help us reflect on our thoughts in general. Thoughts and ensuing emotions are the most powerful sources of stress and are unfortunately the least emphasized and understood phenomena.

Worksheet 2.2
Do You Suffer from Chronic Stress?

Check all the items that apply to you.

____ 1. I frequently suffer from a burning sensation in the upper abdominal region.

____ 2. I often have difficulty digesting food and have belching.

____ 3. I often have backache or joint pains.

____ 4. I frequently suffer from headaches.

____ 5. I sometimes have chest pain.

____ 6. I have been diagnosed as having heart disease or hypertension.

____ 7. I have had a stroke in the past.

____ 8. I frequently develop cold hands and feet.

____ 9. I frequently have diarrhea and loose movements, especially when I am anxious.

____ 10. I suffer from a great deal of anxiety.

FEEDBACK ON WORKSHEET 2.2

If you have checked any of the items, you are likely to be suffering from the effects of chronic stress. Don't worry! It is still not too late to change your lifestyle.

If you have checked items 1 and 2, then you are a likely candidate for a *peptic ulcer,* which is precipitated and aggravated by stress. Item 3 pertains to *backache* and *arthritis,* which have been associated with chronic stress. Item 4 refers to *migraine* and *tension headaches,* which are a result of stress. Items 5–7 pertain to *coronary heart disease* and *hypertension.* Item 8 refers to *circulatory problems,* which are stress related. Item 9 indicates *diarrhea* and *colitis,* which have been related to stress. Finally, Item 10 pertains to generalized anxiety disorder, which is also a result of chronic stress.

If you are young, it is likely that you may not have checked any of the items. This result only indicates that you have not yet been invaded by the harmful effects of stress. Therefore, it is all the more a reason for you to practice stress reduction, prevention, and management techniques.

* * * * *

Worksheet 2.3
Thought Identification

For the next 15 minutes leave aside everything you have been doing and try to write down *all* the thoughts that are coming into your mind in the space provided. Be sure to write down everything, even if it may appear trivial or unimportant.

FEEDBACK ON WORKSHEET 2.3

Notice how many thoughts have come to your mind in such a short period of time—just 15 minutes. Count these thoughts. A multiplication of this figure by four will provide you with the number of thoughts that come to your mind in an hour. Go ahead and calculate the total number of thoughts that come to your mind in a year and in an expected lifetime of 75 years.

Number of thoughts in 15 minutes:		(A) =	_______
Number of thoughts in 1 hour:	(B) =	$(A \times 4)$ =	_______
Number of thoughts in 1 day:	(C) =	$(B \times 24)$ =	_______
Number of thoughts in 1 year:	(D) =	$(C \times 365)$ =	_______
Number of thoughts in 75 years:	(E) =	$(D \times 75)$ =	_______

This is a simplistic calculation. For the sake of simplicity we have included all the time in the day. However, when we are deeply engrossed in certain tasks, or when we are in a deep sleep, the number of thoughts decreases. It needs to be noted that in light sleep, while dreaming, the frequency of thoughts increases. In essence, this pattern may have a canceling-out effect. Therefore, these calculations may be close to accuracy owing to the canceling-out effect.

Thus you can appreciate that in your lifetime you generate a large number of thoughts and that only a few of these are relevant and need to be processed. This approach will help you to reduce your stress and lead a productive life.

* * * * *

Stress and Expectations

All of us will appreciate that the body has only a limited potential to process a few of the thoughts that come to our mind and that most of the unwanted, unprocessed thoughts contribute to our stress levels. Since we cannot do anything about the unwanted, unprocessed thoughts, we need to be selective and judiciously indulge in only those thoughts that we can process. The techniques to reduce these thoughts can only be acquired through proper conditioning of the mind over a period of time. This reduction in the number of unwanted thoughts will most certainly help in reducing our stress levels. How we interpret and label these thoughts is also an important dimension. Imagine a situation in which we observe our boss or teacher looking at us in an unusual way. It is easy for us to attribute to this look the meaning that we are not doing well, and this reaction is likely to be stressful and anxiety provoking. Interpretation of the same event as being due to his or her being tired or having personal problems will not cause stress. Brooding over our thoughts or dwelling on our worries only adds to the tension in our body, which in turn creates the subjective feeling of uneasiness and leads to more anxious thoughts. Becoming excessively emotional about these thoughts is another factor that contributes to stress. Emotions or feelings are helpful, but if we become unduly emotional, then the emotions do not serve any purpose. Instead these emotions do more harm than good by stimulating the physiological processes and precipitating the stress response. This stress response drains away the vital energy needed by the body to perform important daily functions.

Stress is also the result of our interactions with people, situations, and the environment. If we think about people and situations that contribute to our stress, we will find that people who are close to us and situations from which we expect to benefit are the ones that contribute to most of our stress. This stress is tied into the inherent *expectation* that we have of these people and situations. Is this expectation realistic? Most of the time it is not.

We cannot become hermits or renounce the world and escape all stresses of life. However, we can learn to counteract our conventional response to stress by learning how to relax effectively and by reducing unwanted thoughts. These techniques help the body in attaining a state of balance or *homeostasis*. Relaxation and modification of thoughts restore our lost energy. Before we discuss relaxation techniques, effective communication techniques, methods for managing anger, coping with anxiety, maintaining a balanced diet, ways to exercise regularly, and managing time efficiently by modifying our thought process, we have to enhance our awareness of the type, frequency, intensity, and duration of stress operating in our body. An awareness of any problem is certainly the first step toward aiming at a solution. Therefore, it is important for us to begin examining questions pertaining to what, where, how, and when before we begin searching for a solution. The worksheets that follow are aimed at achieving an enhancement of your awareness about stress. You may now complete Worksheets 2.4, 2.5, and 2.6.

Worksheet 2.4
Stress Awareness Log

Principles

A daily record of stressors can serve as a valuable tool in learning to cope with stress. Keeping a stress record through log sheets is an excellent tool for this purpose. The stress awareness log serves three important purposes:

1. It helps to familiarize how you respond to stress.

2. It helps to rule out other than stress-related causes to any symptoms you might have.

3. It helps in establishing some baseline data and developing goals for yourself in reducing stress.

Initially, maintaining this stress awareness log may appear complicated and time-consuming; however, it is not. Once you have used these log sheets for a few days and have become familiar with this means of record keeping, it will take only a few minutes of your time every day.

The information that you record on the stress log sheets is for your use only. You need not share it with anyone. It is important that you be *candid and honest* with yourself in filling out these log sheets. If your daily experiences remain unclear, then the means for finding appropriate solutions will also be hazy. It is important that you maintain the log sheets for *at least four or five consecutive days.* Try to include a weekend in your recordings, as we normally tend to behave differently over weekends and sometimes this difference may result in contributing to your stress.

The most important part of the stress awareness log is for you to maintain it *conscientiously.* It is a very effective tool to help you identify ways in which you respond to stress. However, unless you maintain it accurately and work at it, it will be of no value and may even contribute to increasing your stress levels. The more information you put into this stress awareness log, the more you will benefit from it in the long run.

Recording Instructions

Under the headings listed in the following paragraphs, you should make a record on the log sheets as described.

Time of day includes a serial record of time for each event chronologically. You need to use one log sheet per day. Photocopy the sheet provided in order to record your information for a minimum of four or five days.

Worksheet 2.4 Stress Awareness Log (cont'd)

Signals are indicators, manifestations, signs, symptoms, responses, reactions (e.g., *physical*—headache, muscle tension, perspiration, palpitation, or rapid heart rate; *mental*—loss of attention span, poor concentration, effect on memory, impaired judgment; *behavioral*—inability to interact with others, uncontrolled anger, reduced job performance).

Stressors are events that can be looked upon as "inputs" originating from your thoughts, situations, and the environment. If the event causes stress or interferes with your ability to accomplish daily tasks, then it is a stressor. It is also important to consider different intensity levels of various stressors.

How am I dealing with the stressors? In this section you can record techniques and mechanisms, if any, that you have been using in handling the stressors. It would also be worthwhile to record the time of the day the technique was used. Also record whether or not it made any difference.

How effective have I been? What else can I do? This section would include whether or not you were able to work with the stressor in a satisfactory way and whether or not the means of resolution worked. Other comments, if necessary, may be added in this section.

Now you can begin recording on the sheets for at least four to five consecutive days. You may also prepare a brief summary statement of the information entered on your log sheets, if you need to share it with someone else or if you want concise information from these recordings for greater insight.

Worksheet 2.4 Stress Awareness Log (cont'd)

DAY AND DATE: ______________________________

Time of Day	*Signals*	*Stressor*	*How Am I Dealing with the Stressors?*	*How Effective Have I Been? What Else Can I Do?*

FEEDBACK ON WORKSHEET 2.4

Maintaining a stress awareness log is an excellent tool that provides you with accurate feedback about your present stress levels. If it is maintained carefully and honestly, it generates useful insight into your own behavior that provides an important basis for initiating change in your lifestyle. It also provides you with an opportunity to look at unhealthy lifestyles that are jeopardizing your own health. It is an important first step to initiate any subsequent changes.

In order to interpret the information from the Stress Awareness Log you need to be objective. You need to critically appraise your behavior and identify the changes that can be easily and effectively incorporated into your daily lifestyle. In subsequent chapters of this workbook these changes have been elaborated on step by step.

* * * * *

Worksheet 2.5
Stress and Tension Test

Search your memory of the past month, and try to answer the following questions as honestly as possible. Circle your responses.

	Always	*Often*	*Sometimes*	*Rarely*
1. I feel tense, anxious, and uptight.	3	2	1	0
2. I cannot stop worrying at night, and during my leisure time.	3	2	1	0
3. I have headaches, backache, and pain in the shoulder or neck.	3	2	1	0
4. My sleep is disrupted and I usually keep getting up while sleeping.	3	2	1	0
5. People around me tend to cause me stress and make me irritable.	3	2	1	0
6. I tend to eat, drink, and/or smoke in response to my stress and anxiety.	3	2	1	0
7. I do not feel refreshed in the mornings and am normally tired, lethargic, and exhausted during the day.	3	2	1	0
8. I find it difficult to concentrate on the tasks and activities that I am supposed to perform.	3	2	1	0

Worksheet 2.5 Stress and Tension Test (cont'd)

	Always	*Often*	*Sometimes*	*Rarely*
9. I have to use tranquilizers, sedatives, or other drugs to relax me.	3	2	1	0
10. I do not find time to relax.	3	2	1	0
11. I have too many deadlines to meet, and I fall behind in accomplishing them.	3	2	1	0

Note: From John W. Farquhar, M.D., *The American way of life need not be hazardous to your health,* Revised Edition, © 1987 by the Stanford Alumni Association. Adapted by permission of Addison-Wesley Publishing Company, Inc.

FEEDBACK ON WORKSHEET 2.5

This instrument helps you to reflect on your life during the past month. If you have a score over 22, then you certainly have been having high stress levels, you need to work at getting relaxed by practicing stress management techniques. You may also require help from others. If your score is below 22, then you may not be stressed as much at present, but in order to continue being relaxed and stress free, you need to practice techniques of stress management, reduction, and prevention.

* * * * *

Worksheet 2.6
Personal Stress Test

This test is designed to help you assess the impact of stress at this point in your life. Your response to each statement can provide information to help you deal with stress. This test does not assess physical, mental, or emotional illness. It is designed for normal, healthy individuals who want to control stress in a positive manner and enjoy life more.

Fill out the test when you are certain not to be interrupted. Respond to each statement using the scale at the right side of the page. There are no right or wrong answers. Some statements may seem hard to respond to because they are subjective. If none of the available responses appears to fit perfectly, pick the one closest to the way you feel. You need not consult the test feedback sheet until you have finished the test. While it is not mandatory to respond to any item you find objectionable, results from completed tests are more accurate. Thus you need to complete the entire test.

Circle the letter to the right of each statement that best describes you and how often you feel that way. Answer each statement honestly. If you do not, you are cheating only yourself.

PROFILE CODE: N = almost never; R = rarely; S = sometimes; O = often; A = almost always

PROFILE QUESTIONS:

1. There are situations in which I cannot be myself.	N	R	S	O	A
2. I have the stamina and endurance I need.	N	R	S	O	A
3. I worry about how things will turn out.	N	R	S	O	A
4. I am happy and content.	N	R	S	O	A
5. I feel motivated to do things.	N	R	S	O	A
6. I feel sad and down in the dumps.	N	R	S	O	A
7. I feel in control of my appetite.	N	R	S	O	A
8. I am sluggish and lack energy.	N	R	S	O	A
9. I feel loved by someone important to me.	N	R	S	O	A
10. I feel well organized and clearheaded.	N	R	S	O	A
11. My life lacks stimulation.	N	R	S	O	A
12. Day-to-day living is monotonous for me.	N	R	S	O	A
13. I accomplish things that are important to me.	N	R	S	O	A
14. I feel physically strong and capable.	N	R	S	O	A

Worksheet 2.6 Personal Stress Test (cont'd)

15. I fit in well with the people around me.	N	R	S	O	A
16. I feel resentment about things that have happened to me in the past.	N	R	S	O	A
17. I enjoy being with the people around me.	N	R	S	O	A
18. There is a difference between how I think I should be and how I am.	N	R	S	O	A
19. My stomach bothers me.	N	R	S	O	A
20. I am lonely.	N	R	S	O	A
21. I think I am living to the fullest.	N	R	S	O	A
22. I have the standard of living I deserve.	N	R	S	O	A
23. I feel excluded by people.	N	R	S	O	A
24. I have difficulty concentrating.	N	R	S	O	A
25. I feel relaxed.	N	R	S	O	A
26. I feel guilty about eating.	N	R	S	O	A
27. I have a clear conscience.	N	R	S	O	A
28. I have aches and pains.	N	R	S	O	A
29. I would like to start all over.	N	R	S	O	A
30. I have pleasant feelings.	N	R	S	O	A
31. It is hard for me to get close to people.	N	R	S	O	A
32. I worry about my weight.	N	R	S	O	A
33. I feel I belong.	N	R	S	O	A
34. I feel like I am part of a family.	N	R	S	O	A
35. My life is dull and uninteresting.	N	R	S	O	A
36. Things that happen to me are unfair.	N	R	S	O	A
37. I can remember important things.	N	R	S	O	A
38. I feel nervous or upset.	N	R	S	O	A
39. I feel good about my eating habits.	N	R	S	O	A
40. I get what I want.	N	R	S	O	A

FEEDBACK ON WORKSHEET 2.6

1. Place your Personal Stress Test alongside the following answer key.
2. This answer key is divided into ten categories.

   Note: The order of the items on this answer key is *not* the same as the order on the test.
3. To find the score for each item, carefully circle the number below the letter you chose on your stress test.
4. Enter the score for each question in the proper bracket in the Total Points column.
5. Then total the score for each category on the following page.

FEEDBACK ON WORKSHEET 2.6 (cont'd)

Stress Factor	*Question Number*	*Scoring Key* N	R	S	O	A	*Total Points*
1. Physical condition	2.	5	4	3	2	1	______
	8.	1	2	3	4	5	______
	14.	5	4	3	2	1	______
	28.	1	2	3	4	5	______
					Subtotal		______
2. Mental performance	3.	1	2	3	4	5	______
	10.	5	4	3	2	1	______
	24.	1	2	3	4	5	______
	37.	5	4	3	2	1	______
					Subtotal		______
3. Emotional relaxation	19.	1	2	3	4	5	______
	25.	5	4	3	2	1	______
	30.	5	4	3	2	1	______
	38.	1	2	3	4	5	______
					Subtotal		______
4. Weight control and image	7.	5	4	3	2	1	______
	26.	1	2	3	4	5	______
	32.	1	2	3	4	5	______
	39.	5	4	3	2	1	______
					Subtotal		______
5. Sense of belonging	15.	5	4	3	2	1	______
	20.	1	2	3	4	5	______
	33.	5	4	3	2	1	______
	34.	5	4	3	2	1	______
					Subtotal		______
6. Sense of relationship	9.	5	4	3	2	1	______
	17.	5	4	3	2	1	______
	23.	1	2	3	4	5	______
	31.	1	2	3	4	5	______
					Subtotal		______

FEEDBACK ON WORKSHEET 2.6 (cont'd)

Stress Factor	*Question Number*	*Scoring Key*					*Total Points*
		N	*R*	*S*	*O*	*A*	
7. Sense of satisfaction	4.	5	4	3	2	1	______
	21.	5	4	3	2	1	______
	29.	1	2	3	4	5	______
	35.	1	2	3	4	5	______
					Subtotal		______
8. Sense of integrity	1.	1	2	3	4	5	______
	13.	5	4	3	2	1	______
	18.	1	2	3	4	5	______
	27.	5	4	3	2	1	______
					Subtotal		______
9. Sense of justice	16.	1	2	3	4	5	______
	22.	5	4	3	2	1	______
	36.	1	2	3	4	5	______
	40.	5	4	3	2	1	______
					Subtotal		______
10. Sense of stimulation	5.	5	4	3	2	1	______
	6.	1	2	3	4	5	______
	11.	1	2	3	4	5	______
	12.	1	2	3	4	5	______
					Subtotal		______

Now transfer these scores where indicated on the following sheet to obtain your Personal Stress Profile.

FEEDBACK ON WORKSHEET 2.6 (cont'd)

Transfer the subtotal scores calculated on the preceding page for each category under the subtotal scores column below. Then place an X on the adjoining scale. This scale visually reveals your areas of low, moderate, and high stress in these categories.

Personal Stress Profile:

		SCALE					
		Low		*Moderate*		*High*	
Stress Profile Factor	*Subtotal Scores*	*0*	*4*	*8*	*12*	*16*	*20*
1. Physical condition	______						
2. Mental performance	______						
3. Emotional relaxation	______						
4. Weight control and image	______						
5. Sense of belonging	______						
6. Sense of relationship	______						
7. Sense of satisfaction	______						
8. Sense of integrity	______						
9. Sense of justice	______						
10. Sense of stimulation	______						

FEEDBACK ON WORKSHEET 2.6 (cont'd)

Interpretation of Scores:

	COMMON INDICATORS		
Factor	*High 12–20 (Poor Coping)*	*Moderate 9–11 (Dissatisfaction)*	*Low 4–8 (Good Coping)*
1. Physical condition	• Aches, pains • Fatigue • Listlessness • Illness prone	• Energy level fluctuations • Little stamina	• Stamina • Strength • Active
2. Mental performance	• Forgets details • Worries a lot • Ruminates	• Confusion • Mind vacillates • Details escape	• Clarity • Solves problems • Concentrate
3. Emotional relaxation	• Tense • Nervous • Anxious • Sleeplessness • Stomach churnings	• Irritable • Inner turmoil • Some tension	• Calm • Confident • Relaxed
4. Weight control and image	• Eats more • Disappointed with image	• Eats too much or too little • Not satisfied with image	• Eats when hungry • Balanced diet
5. Sense of belonging	• Alienated • Loneliness • Separation	• Close to only a few • Distant with others	• Common bonds with many • Comfortable with others
6. Sense of relation	• Tense relations • Withdrawal	• Shares little about self • Few inquiries about others • Unpredictable	• Strong friendships • Long-term relations

FEEDBACK ON WORKSHEET 2.6 (cont'd)

Interpretation of Scores:

	COMMON INDICATORS		
Factor	*High 12–20 (Poor Coping)*	*Moderate 9–11 (Dissatisfaction)*	*Low 4–8 (Good Coping)*
7. Sense of satisfaction	• Wanting to start life over	• Unsure • Questions • Disinterested • Discontent	• Happy • Contented • Enthusiasm • Fulfillment
8. Sense of integrity	• Reserved • Unsure • Expedient	• Inconsistent • Regrets behavior • Attitude of martyrdom	• Acts on priorities • Pride in accomplishment
9. Sense of justice	• Resentment • Anger • Incapable	• Roll with punches • Questions	• Control • Fairness • Balance
10. Sense of stimulation	• Monotony • Boredom • Laziness	• Moderate interest in life • Future has appeal	• Enthusiasm • Motivation • Takes initiative

Note: From *Coping with stress* by Medicine Shoppe International, Inc., 1985, St. Louis, MO: Medicine Shoppe International, Inc. Copyright 1985 Medicine Shoppe International, Inc. Adapted by permission. All Rights Reserved. May not be reproduced without permission of Medicine Shoppe International, Inc.

* * * * *

Thoughts for Reflection 2.1
Commitment

- Is it not true that commitment is vital to the success of any task?
- Imagine all your past successes. Were you not committed to the tasks?
- Does commitment not reduce stress?
- If you are committed, would that fact not reduce the chances of self-doubt, failure, and inefficiency? Would that improvement not in turn reduce stress?
- What if you are not committed? Would that fact not add to the confusion of roles that you perform? Would your confusion not contribute to purposelessness and lack of direction?

* * * * *

Thoughts for Reflection 2.2
True Happiness or *Ananda*

True happiness or *ananda* only arises if we focus on the present. If we can be happy now, then we have learned to be happy anytime. However, if we choose to believe that we will be happy . . .

- if . . .
- when . . .
- with . . .
- only if . . .
- in . . .

then we are only making our happiness contingent on external things. We may become happy temporarily, but true happiness will elude us. True happiness or *ananda* is an internal feeling that cannot be dependent on any external object. This understanding has to be appreciated by us and also implemented in our daily life. We have to constantly keep reminding ourselves that true happiness or *ananda* is an internal phenomenon not dependent on the outside world. We have to learn to be happy, . . . "just happy" and not happy . . . "due to."

* * * * *

Stress Management Principle 2

You need to become aware before considering change.

Summary Points

- For any change to occur besides knowledge, enhanced awareness is essential.
- Components of the Health Belief Model, which explains and predicts behavior change, are perceived susceptibility, perceived severity, perceived benefits, perceived barriers, cues to action, and self-efficacy.
- Stress affects all of us. We all experience acute and chronic manifestations of stress.
- The acute manifestations of stress present themselves either predominantly in the body, or primarily in the mind. For some, there may be a mixed reaction on both the body and mind.
- Diseases like hypertension, coronary heart disease, stroke, migraine headaches, peptic ulcers, arthritis, colitis, diarrhea, asthma, cardiac arrhythmias, sexual problems, circulatory problems, muscle tension, allergies, backache, temporomandibular joint syndrome, and cancer have been found to be associated with stress.
- Maintaining a daily observation of the stress in our lives is the first and foremost step in dealing with stress.
- Commitment to alleviating stress is a vital prerequisite for initiating stress management programs.

References and Further Readings

Bandura, A. (Ed.). (1995). *Self-efficacy in changing societies.* New York: Cambridge University Press.

Becker, M. H. (1974). The health belief model and personal health behavior. *Health Education Monographs, 2,* 324–473.

Farquhar, J. W. (1979). *The American way of life need not be hazardous to your health.* New York: W. W. Norton.

Girdano, D. A., Everly, G. S., Jr., & Dusek, D. E. (1997). *Controlling stress and tension: A holistic approach* (5th ed.). Englewood Cliffs, NJ: Prentice Hall.

Glanz, K., Lewis, F. M., & Rimer, B. K. (1997). *Health behavior and health education: Theory, Research, and Practice* (2nd ed.). San Francisco: Jossey-Bass.

Green, L. W., & Kreuter, M. W. (1991). *Health promotion planning: An educational and environmental approach* (2nd ed.). Mountain View, CA: Mayfield.

Greenberg, J. S. (1999). *Comprehensive stress management* (6th ed.). Boston: William C. Brown/McGraw-Hill.

Hochbaum, G. M. (1958). *Public participation in medical screening programs: A sociopsychological study.* PHS Publication No. 572. Washington, DC: U.S. Government Printing Office.

Labarthe, D. R., & Roccella, E. J. (1993). High blood pressure. In R. C. Brownson, P. L. Remington, & J. R. Davis (Eds.), *Chronic disease epidemiology and control* (p. 109). Washington, DC: American Public Health Association.

Rice, P. L. (1999). *Stress and health* (3rd ed.). Pacific Grove, CA: Brooks/Cole.

Smith, J. C. (1993). *Understanding stress and coping.* New York: Macmillan.

CHAPTER 3

Relaxation

Sleep

Come, Sleep! O Sleep, the certain knot of peace,
The baiting-place of wit, the balm of woe,
The poor man's wealth, the prisoner's release,
Th' indifferent judge between the high and low.

—Sir Philip Sidney
(Astrophel and Stella, Sonnet 39)

What Is Relaxation?

The word "relax" is derived from the Latin word *relaxare* meaning to loosen. Indeed relaxation implies loosening up or letting go. By this process of relaxing or loosening, all living beings consolidate and restore energy that has been lost in daily activities. Therefore, relaxation is vital for the normal functioning of any living organism. Relaxation techniques form the core of all stress management programs. When our bodies are functioning normally, we derive relaxation through sleep.

Sleep

We all sleep. Without sleep we cannot live, although there may be some exceptions. Sleep accomplishes two vital functions—conservation of energy and restoration of energy (Shapiro & Flanigan, 1993). Expenditure of energy is mainly measured by the metabolic rate (in simple terms, the rate of conversion of ingested food into energy useful for the body), which is raised during the day and reduced during the night (particularly during sleep) by between 5 percent and 25 percent (Shapiro & Flanigan, 1993). Physiologically, sleep is composed of two phases:

1. *Non-REM (Non–Rapid Eye Movement) sleep*
   The non-REM sleep phase is characterized by four stages:

   - *Stage 1* is a light, drowsy phase of non-REM sleep (the transition from wakefulness to sleep). Electroencephalography is a scientific method that helps to gauge the electrical impulses within the brain with the help of electrodes placed over the scalp. Normally, if this electroencephalogram (EEG) recording is done during the awake state, when our mind and senses are working, then this recording will manifest beta waves (fast waves at a rhythm of 14 to 40 cycles per second). As drowsiness sets in, the frequency of beta waves starts to recede.

• *Stage 2* is the first real stage of sleep, which is characterized by "spindles" and "K complexes" on an EEG. During this stage of non-REM sleep, the EEG will record alpha waves (slower waves at 8–13 cycles per second). In this stage, the mind comes to a peaceful state.

• *Stages 3 and 4* are known as "slow wave sleep." In these stages of non-REM-phase sleep the mind gets subtler, and the EEG records theta waves (4–7 cycles per second). In extremely deep sleep or coma, the EEG records delta waves (near 1 cycle per second).

2. *REM (Rapid Eye Movement) sleep*

REM sleep is the phase during which most dreaming happens. It occurs approximately 90 minutes after the person falls asleep. During this stage the mind functions at alpha and beta waves. From a stress perspective, during this phase a person does not actually get relaxed. However, this is still an important phase of sleep.

There is a cycle of non-REM and REM sleep throughout the night. As the night progresses, the episodes of non-REM sleep become shorter, and those of the REM phase of sleep longer. Most slow-wave sleep occurs during the first third of the night, and most REM sleep during the last third of sleep (Kalat, 1988).

However, when we are stressed, our normal biorhythm is altered and our sleep pattern is disturbed. Therefore, our bodies are not able to conserve and restore the lost energy. This lack in turn adds to the stress, and a vicious cycle is set up. If this disturbed sleep pattern is not changed or relaxation methods are not used, complete balance and harmony are disrupted.

It may even be the other way around. If, for reasons of overwork or not being able to find enough time, we sleep less, our biorhythm gets altered. Therefore, the body needs other forms of relaxation in order to conserve and restore lost energy.

Relaxation Techniques

Relaxation techniques provide us with excellent methods that can be practiced with awareness at our discretion anytime. This is especially important when we are just beginning to experience stress. In this case, most of the negative consequences of stress can be counteracted even before they have occurred.

Various techniques have been suggested in order to achieve relaxation. In this workbook the methods of Yogic breathing, progressive muscle relaxation, autogenic training, and visual imagery will be described in detail. Other techniques of relaxation such as Yoga, meditation, and biofeedback are also introduced in this workbook. However, these methods require personal instruction and supervision by a qualified and experienced person. Thus the actual techniques for these methods have not been completely elaborated, and the reader is provided with the appropriate resources for obtaining further assistance.

Box 3.1 Yoga and Meditation

Fundamentally, relaxation techniques owe their origin to Eastern cultures, particularly India. They are a part of the overall system of "Yoga" that originated from the *Vedas*. The word "Yoga" is derived from the Sanskrit root meaning "union," implying the joining or yoking of human consciousness to the Divine Being. According to *Webster's New World Dictionary* (1991), Yoga is a mystic and ascetic Hindu discipline by which one seeks to achieve liberation of the self and union with the supreme spirit or universal soul through intense concentration, deep meditation, and practices involving prescribed postures, controlled breathing, and so on. It is a complete system of physical, mental, social, and spiritual development of the human being. A contemporary description of Yoga is "a systematic practice and implementation of mind and body in the living process of human beings to keep harmony within self, within society, and with nature" (Maharishi, 1986, 1987, 1989).

For generations this philosophy was passed on from the master teacher to the student. The first written records about this methodology appeared around 200 B.C. in *Yogasutra* of Patanjali. It was known as *Asthangayoga* or the eightfold path of physical, psychological, and moral discipline, which if properly adhered to, under the guidance of a qualified teacher, results in enhancement of purity and improved stress-coping skills (Singh, 1983). This eightfold path of *Asthangayoga* consists of the following:

1. *Yama:* Restraints or rules for living in society—for example, truthfulness, noninjury, nonstealing, etc.
2. *Niyama:* Observances or rules for self—for example, contentment, cleanliness, etc.
3. *Asaana:* Physical exercises
4. *Pranayama:* Regulated breathing practice
5. *Pratihara:* Detaching the mind from senses
6. *Dharana:* Concentration on an object (internal or external)
7. *Dhyana:* Meditation
8. *Samadhi:* Deep meditation on the cosmic level

This process involves arousal of the *Kundalini Shakti*, or serpent power, believed to be located at the base of the human spine. As the practitioner practices the various techniques, this power rises through a series of centers or *Chakras* corresponding to various endocrine glands. When this power reaches

Box 3.1 Yoga and Meditation (cont'd)

the highest center, *Sahasrara,* which is associated with the hypothalamus gland regulating the hormonal secretion of the endocrine glands, control over the hypothalamus results. In this way secretion of hormones from various endocrine glands can be regulated. This mechanism could possibly explain the important role that this method plays in coping with stress.

In the past Yoga was a very strict and tedious process and was confined to only a select few. However, later many teachers modified the techniques and various paths emerged, like *Bhakti Yoga,* the path of devotion; *Gyana Yoga,* the path of knowledge; *Raja Yoga,* the path of wisdom to self-realization and enlightenment; and *Karma Yoga,* the path of action. Various intermediary techniques like *Hatha Yoga, Mudra Yoga,* and *Chakra Yoga* have also gained popularity.

The system of Yoga is in the process of developing as a science. Various techniques of Yoga have developed and become popular all over the world, particularly in the West, which are, in comparison to the old methods, more simple. Examples of prevalent systems in the West include Transcendental Meditation (TM), *Kriya Yoga,* and Simplified Kundalini Yoga (SKY).

Transcendental Meditation (TM) was developed by Maharishi Mahesh Yogi, disciple of Brahmananda Saraswati, in the year 1957. In 1971 he founded the Maharishi International University in Fairfield, Iowa. In 1975 he established the International Capital of the Age of Enlightenment at Seelisberg in Switzerland, which has now been renamed Maharishi European Research University. TM is a simple, natural technique that can be learned by any person belonging to any age, education, occupation, or cultural background. It has to be practiced every day for 15 to 20 minutes and requires personal instruction by a qualified master who can gauge normal progress and take care of any adverse experiences if they arise. The centers teaching this technique are established all over the world, and the process consists of the following seven steps (Kumar, 1993):

1. Introductory lecture—a vision of the possibilities through TM (60 minutes)
2. Preparatory lecture—the origin and mechanics of TM (60 minutes)
3. Personal interview with the teacher (15 minutes)
4. Personal instruction—learning the technique (60 minutes)
5. Verification and validation of experiences—verifying the correctness of the practice (90 minutes)
6. Understanding the mechanics of stabilizing the benefits of TM (90 minutes)
7. Understanding the mechanics of development of higher states of consciousness through TM (90 minutes)

Box 3.1 Yoga and Meditation (cont'd)

Further information about Transcendental Meditation can be obtained from the Transcendental Meditation National Center, 13039 Ventura Boulevard, Los Angeles, CA 90024, (213) 463–8970.

Kriya Yoga became popular in the West due to the efforts of Paramhansa Yogananda, who founded the Yogoda Satsanga Society in India and the Self-Realization Fellowship in the United States of America. The word *Kriya* is derived from the Sanskrit root *kri* meaning "to do," "to act," and "to react." This method of *Kriya Yoga* involves a psychophysiological method by which human blood is decarbonated and recharged with oxygen. This extra oxygen is converted into life current to rejuvenate the central nervous system, lessen and prevent the decay of tissues, and enhance evolution of the mind (Yogananda, 1946). Further information on this technique and system can be obtained from Self-Realization Fellowship, 3880 San Rafael Avenue, Los Angeles, CA 90065.

A better and more refined system is Yogiraj Vethathiri Maharishi's **Simplified Kundalini Yoga (SKY)**. Yogiraj Vethathiri Maharishi formed the World Community Service Center in 1958. This system was developed as a result of many years of extensive practice and research (Maharishi, 1986, 1987, 1989). It involves the arousal, awakening, and development of *Kundalini Shakti,* which lies dormant in most individuals at *Mooladhara,* at the base of the spine. The energy levels are raised to *Agna Chakra* and then to *Sahasrara.* The important aspect of this system is *Shanti Yoga,* which helps keep control of the powerful awakened *Kundalini Shakti.* Other important aspects of this system include simplified physical exercises; introspection, or analysis of thoughts (as described in Chapter 6); and *Kaya Kalpa* which is a system of exercises designed to improve upon health and longevity. Interested readers can contact the organization headquarters at the following addresses: World Community Service Center, 20 Second Seaward Street, Valmiki Nagar, Thiruvanmiyur, Madras 600 041, India, or in the United States at World Community Service Center of California, 926 La Rambla, Burbank, CA 91501, (818) 848–1509; Toma and Adele Fitzgerald, 12205 Gorham, No. 4, Brentwood, CA 90049, (310) 207–4871; Ram Patil, 9343 Larch, Munster, IN 46321, (219) 924–6301; Dr. M. Sharma, 4311 South 150th Street, Omaha, NE 68137, (402) 896-4205.

Other systems of meditation include (Naranjo & Ornstein, 1971):

- *Soto Zen,* which involves focusing on external objects,
- *Rinzai Zen,* in which the mind has to focus on koans (unanswerable, illogical riddles),
- *Zazen,* in which the mind has to focus on subjective states of consciousness, and
- *Tibetan Meditation,* in which the mind has to focus on geometrical figures.

* * * * *

Yogic Breathing or *Pranayama*

All of us breathe. Breathing is a vital function for life. However, we seldom pay attention to how we breathe. This is an important aspect of life and needs to be understood. The process of breathing has received special emphasis in the system of Yoga. As mentioned earlier, this process is known as *Pranayama.* The purpose of this technique is not only to increase the vital capacity of the lungs, but also to enhance the oxygenation capacity of the blood by the lungs. The oxygen from the air that we breathe in is carried by the hemoglobin in the blood to the various parts of the body for providing energy. If greater oxygen can be carried by the blood, then greater restoration of energy that has been lost in daily activities can be achieved. Therefore, the process of Yogic breathing or *Pranayama* is essential for achieving relaxation and managing stress. In simple terms, Yogic breathing consists of three stages (Vasu, 1915):

- *Puraka* (inhalation)
- *Kumbhaka* (pausing or holding the breath)
- *Rechaka* (exhalation)

The ratio of these three stages is 1 : 4 : 2—that is, if one inhales the air for four seconds, then the person has to hold the air for sixteen seconds, and then exhale the air over a period of eight seconds. The purpose of Yogic breathing or *Pranayama* is to achieve this kind of rhythmic breathing. We sometimes achieve this kind of breathing pattern when we are engrossed in some task with deep concentration, or some of us may be naturally gifted with this kind of pattern. This type of breathing pattern helps the body to relax and conserve energy. It has been found to be useful in curing chronic muscle fatigue, migraine and tension headaches, and other stress-related disorders. Worksheet 3.1 is based upon the traditional basic principles of Yogic breathing but has been slightly modified to make it feasible for modern times and give it universal applicability. Women, however, are advised not to follow this technique during the course of pregnancy and the postpartum period, because it may cause unwanted pressure and/or hormonal changes that may affect the growing fetus.

Thoughts for Reflection 3.1 will help you to reflect upon some of the barriers that may be hindering you from getting enough relaxation.

Thoughts for Reflection 3.1
Barriers to Relaxation

Reflect upon the following barriers that might be hindering your path to relaxing effectively.

- *Working Long Hours.* Some of us, in our quest to earn greater material wealth or for other reasons, may be working more than is normally required. As a result, we may have less time to relax.

- *Brooding.* Repetitive thinking of the same thoughts over and over again is brooding. It is often counterproductive. It is a barrier to relaxation.

- *Unchecked Imagination.* If we do not put a restriction on our imagination, then we may generate thousands of ideas in a short time that are an important barrier to relaxation.

- *Heavy Meals.* Eating more than required for maintaining the functioning of your body often results in indigestion. It also liberates greater energy. These factors hinder effective relaxation.

- *Inefficient Time Management.* Planning your time well is very important. If you do not provide yourself with adequate time for relaxation, you will not be able to relax properly.

- *Not Enough Faith in the Power of Relaxation.* It is essential for any method to be really effective that it command respect and faith from those utilizing it. Some of us do not have enough faith in the power of relaxation. This lack of faith colors our perspective and prevents us from getting complete relaxation.

* * * * *

Worksheet 3.1
Yogic Breathing or *Pranayama*

You can practice Yogic breathing at any time, but you should not have taken food over the previous two hours. The best time to perform this technique is early morning on an empty stomach or evening before supper. Pregnant women should *not* do this during the course of their pregnancy or immediate postpartum period.

A. Basic Breathing

Step 1. Sit down in a relaxed posture. The ideal posture is squatting with the legs crossed. Place a watch in front of yourself.

Step 2. Inhale deeply and slowly. As you inhale, fill your lungs completely, starting from the lower section to the middle, and proceeding to the upper section. Mentally record the time of completing the inhalation. Usually for beginners this time could range anywhere from four to sixteen seconds. With practice this time can be increased. Though, traditionally, there is no limit to the time, we would recommend that you not exceed twenty seconds for the process of inhalation without supervision from an experienced practitioner.

Step 3. Hold your breath for a duration of four times the amount of time that you had taken for completing the inhalation.

Step 4. Exhale the air slowly in a time that is twice the time you had taken to complete inhaling or half the time you had taken in holding the breath.

Step 5. Repeat Steps 3–5 five times over the first week. Then gradually increase the number of times over a period of the next few months. We would recommend that repetitions in one sitting not exceed fifty and that not more than two sessions a day be performed at that level without supervision from an experienced practitioner.

B. Bending Breathing

Step 1. Kneel down or stand up straight.

Step 2. Inhale slowly and completely. First fill the lower section of the lungs, then the middle, and finally the upper section.

Step 3. While bending down from your original position, gradually exhale the air completely. You may take approximately the same amount of time that you took for inhaling.

Worksheet 3.1 Yogic Breathing or *Pranayama* (cont'd)

Step 4. While rising up from your original position, gradually inhale and fill your lungs completely.

Step 5. Repeat Steps 3–4 five times for the first week. Then gradually increase your frequency over the next couple of months. Again we would recommend a maximum of twenty times twice a day.

C. Alternative Breathing

Step 1. Sit in a comfortable position.

Step 2. Close your right nostril with the thumb of your right hand.

Step 3. Inhale air slowly and completely through your left nostril.

Step 4. Exhale air slowly and completely through your left nostril.

Step 5. Repeat Steps 2–4 five times.

Step 6. Close your left nostril with the index and middle fingers of your right hand.

Step 7. Inhale air slowly and completely through your right nostril.

Step 8. Exhale air slowly and completely through your right nostril.

Step 9. Repeat Steps 6–8 five times.

Step 10. In this step you should practice alternative breathing. Close your right nostril with your right thumb and inhale air slowly and completely through your left nostril. As soon as you complete inhalation, close your left nostril with the index and middle fingers of your right hand. Exhale air through the right nostril.

Step 11. Repeat Step 10 five times.

Step 12. Close your left nostril with the index and middle fingers of your right hand. Inhale air slowly and completely through your right nostril. As soon as you complete inhalation, close your right nostril with the thumb of your right hand. Exhale air through your left nostril.

Step 13. Repeat Step 12 five times.

FEEDBACK ON WORKSHEET 3.1

Yogic breathing is a practice-based technique that has to be done regularly. You may do it once a day or two times. You need not exceed the maximal frequency. This is a useful technique, which if practiced regularly can modify the conventional fight-or-flight response to stress and reduce undue anxiety. Once you have mastered the Yogic breathing technique, it can also be easily practiced to relieve stress. All you need to do is sit down and perform Yogic breathing whenever you are stressed. A couple of breaths taken in will rechannelize the response and reduce the negative stimulation associated with stress.

* * * * *

Biofeedback

Biofeedback has been defined as the use of instrumentation to mirror psychological processes of which the individual is not normally aware and which may be brought under voluntary control (Brown, 1974; Fuller, 1977; Karlins & Andrews, 1972). The primary objective of biofeedback is monitoring and modification of the psychophysiological response that is obtained by enhancing awareness of internal states connected with deep levels of relaxation. Usually, information about internal vital functions such as blood pressure, heart rhythm, muscle tension, and so on is electronically recorded. This information is then explained to the participant, who is then encouraged to work gradually at modifying the responses by exerting greater relaxation. Gradually the participant is enabled to gain greater modifying power on these internal functions that contribute to the reduction of stress. Biofeedback is normally administered with the help of a therapist. Sessions of one hour each last anywhere from 10 to 40 in number. The process involves three phases:

- Measurement of the psychophysiological parameters
- Conversion of these parameters into simple, understandable forms
- Feedback of this information to the participant

Some of the instruments utilized in biofeedback laboratories are the *electromyograph (EMG),* which measures muscle tension and relaxation; *thermal units,* which measure skin surface temperature; the *electroencephalograph (EEG),* which measures brain wave activity monitored from sensors placed on the scalp; and *galvanic skin response (GSR) units,* which measure sympathetic nervous system changes by recording the changes in sweat response on the skin's surface. Some of the conditions that have been found to be responsive to biofeedback include phobias, anxiety, hypertension, bruxism, asthma, headaches, insomnia, circulatory problems like Raynaud's disease, muscle spasms, and temporomandibular joint syndrome (Stoyva & Budzynski, 1993). The chief advantages of biofeedback practice are the following (Greenberg, 1999):

- A greater control over the body and mind for the participant
- A useful tool for psychologists to monitor bodily reactions to various stressors
- An improvement in self-reliance of the participant in coping with stress

A simple form of biofeedback can be obtained with the help of *biodots.* Biodots are small circular, microencapsulated cholesteric liquid crystals measuring a broad thermal range. In simple terms they can be called miniature thermometers that provide a measurement of skin temperature. These are used as a very general indicator of skin temperature variance. Biodots are designed to be triggered at a temperature over 87° F. Biodots are a versatile and economical tool for persons trained to thermal responses. Biodots are an ideal, yet affordable, device for an introductory example to persons unfamiliar with the most general biofeedback techniques. A biodot can be applied to almost any part of the body. However, the most ideal location is the gentle dip of the juncture between the thumb and the forefinger (Figure 3.1). This site provides the participant with a constant

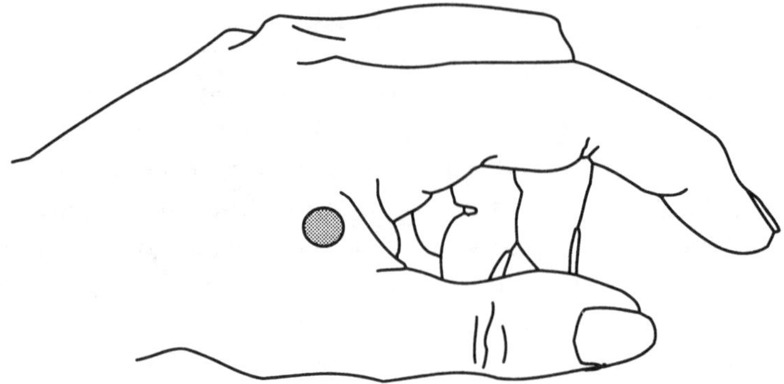

Figure 3.1 Site of Biodot Application

view of the biodot for the purposes of monitoring color change. It is necessary to remember that biodots are the simplest form of biofeedback, and therefore a great amount of trade-off has to be taken into account in terms of their accuracy. Biodots may not be able to provide accurate color change for many of us, especially for those of us who typically have cold hands.

Biodots can be purchased from Biodot International, P.O. Box 2246, Indianapolis, IN 46206, (317) 637–5776. The various color changes that these biodots undergo are depicted in Table 3.1. For more information about Biofeedback the reader can contact the Biofeedback Society of America, Department of Psychiatry C-268, University of Colorado Medical Center, 4200 East Ninth Avenue, Denver, CO 80220.

Table 3.1 Color Changes on Biodots and Their Interpretations

Color	*Temperature*	*Interpretation*
Black	87.5° F	• Indicative of highly tense moment • Normal initial color of the biodot
Amber	89.6° F	• Indicative of tense moment
Yellow	90.6° F	• Unsettled
Green	91.6° F	• Involved with the things going on around the person
Turquoise	92.6° F	• Starting to relax
Blue	93.6° F	• Calm
Violet	94.6° F	• Very relaxed

Progressive Muscle Relaxation

Progressive muscle relaxation was first described by a Chicago physician, Edmund Jacobson (1938, 1977). Jacobson designed this technique for hospital patients who were tense before surgery. He observed that these patients exhibited tenseness of small muscle groups like the ones located in the back or neck and were thus unable to relax. Therefore, he taught these patients to first contract a set of muscles to experience tension and then gradually relax them. This process enabled the individual to discriminate between a relaxed and a tense state. This process was repeated for all other muscle groups throughout the body. The skeletal muscles in the body, which are arranged in various groups, number 1,030. All these muscles can be relaxed by progressive muscle relaxation practiced to cover one group of muscles at a time. This method has been found to be an excellent means by which to achieve relaxation of not only the body confined to skeletal muscles but also the mind and other internal organs. The primary feature of this method is the ability acquired by the practitioner to be able to selectively relax his or her muscle fibers on command, and this can then be done anytime (McGuigan, 1993). Jacobson spent over seven decades collecting data documenting the effectiveness of progressive muscle relaxation in a scientific manner. This method has been shown to have application as a prophylactic method to reduce stress and tension. It also has applicability as a therapeutic measure. Its efficacy has been studied in nervous hypertension, acute insomnia with nervousness, anxiety neurosis, cardiac neurosis, chronic insomnia, cyclothymic depression, compulsive neurosis, hypochondria, fatigue states, nervous depression, and phobias. It has also been successfully applied to somatoform disorders like convulsive tic, esophageal spasm, mucus colitis, chronic colitis, arterial hypertension, and tension headaches (McGuigan, 1993). Bernstein and Carlson (1993) describe another shorter version of PMR known as abbreviated progressive relaxation training (APRT). Attempts to shorten the process of PMR were initiated by Joseph Wolpe (1958), whose method focused on relaxing several major muscle groups in seven sessions in contrast to Jacobson's program, which focused on a single muscle group for several sessions before moving on to the next. This shorter version was further modified by Paul (1966) and formalized by Bernstein and Borkovec (1973). We have, in this workbook, described a modification of all these methods that also include some ideas from Eastern thought. You may now practice this method with the help of Worksheet 3.2.

Thoughts for Reflection 3.2 will help you to ponder appropriate modifications of some of your lifestyles that can provide you with greater relaxation and harmony in life.

Thoughts for Reflection 3.2
Think!

Before going to bed every day, think . . .

- Did I work less, enough, or more? If less or more, then contemplate why.
- Am I getting enough relaxation?
- Is there anything about my lifestyle that I need to change?

Before beginning any new task or activity, think . . .

- Is it worth all the effort?
- Is there any other way to do it better?
- Will it be beneficial to self, family, and society?
- Can I do something else more beneficial in the same time?

Before owning any new object, think . . .

- Do I really need it?
- Is it worth owning?
- What will be the consequences if I own this object?
- What will be the consequences if I do *not* own this object?
- Will it bring happiness and peace to all?

Note: Based upon Eastern philosophy to obtain relaxation and peace.

* * * * *

Worksheet 3.2
Progressive Muscle Relaxation

The method described is a slight modification of the classical approach as advocated by Edmund Jacobson (1938, 1977). The original method takes a longer time, requires greater practice, and is slightly more tedious. This method is a simplification of the classical approach and also incorporates the relaxation component of the physical exercises advocated in Simplified Kundalini Yoga (SKY) as described earlier (Maharishi, 1987).

Preparation

- Seek out a relatively quiet, distraction-free environment, where the practice can be continued for 30 minutes without any interruptions (telephone, doorbell, people entering the room, etc.).
- You need to avoid any unnecessary movements (getting up, fidgeting, etc.) during this process.
- This technique is best practiced in a lying-down supine position with arms placed alongside the body and eyes closed (Figure 3.2).

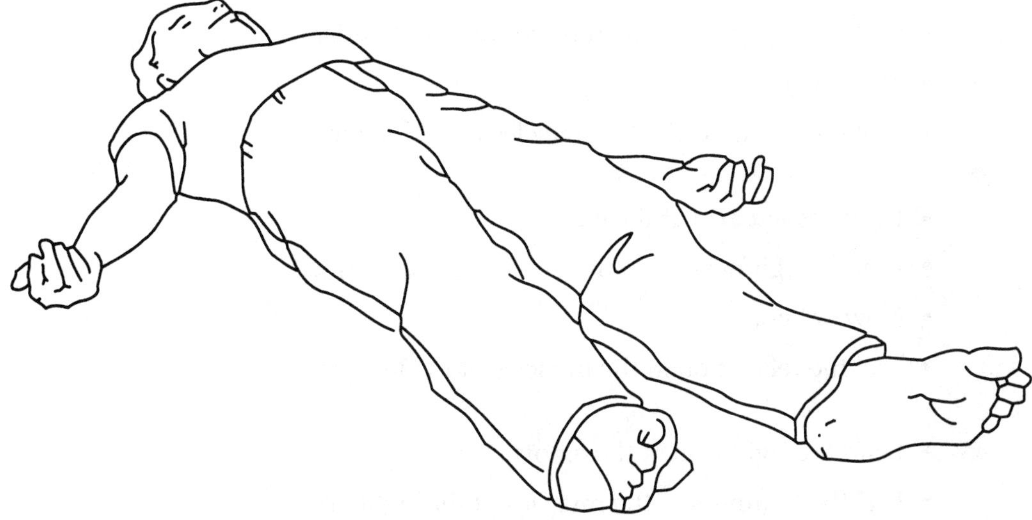

Figure 3.2 Position for Practicing Progressive Muscle Relaxation

Practice Session

You may want to record the following steps in your own voice on a tape recorder, or you may ask another person to record these instructional steps for you. Some people prefer to just repeat the instructions mentally. This approach may require familiarity with these steps, which can be gained by reading them two or three times.

Worksheet 3.2 Progressive Muscle Relaxation (cont'd)

Step 1. **Relaxation of the Arms (6 minutes)**

- Clench the left fist.
- Feel the tightness in the muscles of the left hand.
- Now, let go.
- Feel the relaxation in the muscles of the left hand.

- Clench the right fist.
- Feel the tightness in the muscles of the right hand.
- Now, let go.
- Feel the relaxation in the muscles of the right hand.

- Clench both fists together.
- Feel the tightness in the muscles of both hands.
- Now, let go.
- Feel the relaxation in the muscles of both hands.

- Bend the left arm at the elbow.
- Feel the tightness in the muscles of the left arm.
- Now, let go.
- Feel the relaxation in the muscles of the left arm.

- Bend the right arm at the elbow.
- Feel the tightness in the muscles of the right arm.
- Now, let go.
- Feel the relaxation in the muscles of the right arm.

- Bend both arms at the elbow.
- Feel the tightness in the muscles of both arms.
- Now, let go.
- Feel the relaxation in the muscles of both arms.

Worksheet 3.2 Progressive Muscle Relaxation (cont'd)

Step **2. Relaxation of the Legs (7 minutes)**

- Bend the left foot upward.
- Feel the tightness in the muscles of the left foot
- Now, let go.
- Feel the relaxation in the muscles of the left foot.

- Bend the left foot downward.
- Feel the tightness in the muscles of the left foot.
- Now, let go.
- Feel the relaxation in the muscles of the left foot.

- Bend the right foot upward.
- Feel the tightness in the muscles of the right foot.
- Now, let go.
- Feel the relaxation in the muscles of the right foot.

- Bend the right foot downward.
- Feel the tightness in the muscles of the right foot.
- Now, let go.
- Feel the relaxation in the muscles of the right foot.

- Bend the left leg at the knee and tighten.
- Feel the tightness in the muscles of the left leg and thigh.
- Now, let go.
- Feel the relaxation in the muscles of the left leg and thigh.

- Bend the right leg at the knee and tighten.
- Feel the tightness in the muscles of the right leg and thigh.
- Now, let go.
- Feel the relaxation in the muscles of the right leg and thigh.

- Bend both legs at the knee and tighten.
- Feel the tightness in the muscles of both legs and thighs.

Worksheet 3.2 Progressive Muscle Relaxation (cont'd)

- Now, let go.
- Feel the relaxation in the muscles of both legs and thighs.

Step 3. **Relaxation of the Face (5 minutes)**

- Place wrinkles on the forehead by lifting the eyebrows.
- Feel the tightness in the muscles of the forehead.
- Now, let go.
- Feel the relaxation in the muscles of the forehead.

- Frown by drooping the eyebrows.
- Feel the tightness in the surrounding muscles.
- Now, let go.
- Feel the relaxation in the surrounding muscles.

- Close both eyes tightly shut.
- Feel the tightness in the surrounding muscles.
- Now, let go.
- Feel the relaxation in the surrounding muscles.

- Clench the jaw tightly.
- Feel the tightness in the surrounding muscles.
- Now, let go.
- Feel the relaxation in the surrounding muscles.

- Purse the lips tightly.
- Feel the tightness in the surrounding muscles.
- Now, let go.
- Feel the relaxation in the surrounding muscles.

Step 4. **Relaxation of the Neck and Shoulders (6 minutes)**

- Bend the neck gently forward.
- Feel the tightness in the muscles of the neck.

Worksheet 3.2 Progressive Muscle Relaxation (cont'd)

- Now, let go.
- Feel the relaxation in the muscles of the neck.

- Bend the neck gently backward.
- Feel the tightness in the muscles of the neck.
- Now, let go.
- Feel the relaxation in the muscles of the neck.

- Bend the neck gently to the right.
- Feel the tightness in the muscles of the neck.
- Now, let go.
- Feel the relaxation in the muscles of the neck.

- Bend the neck gently to the left.
- Feel the tightness in the muscles of the neck.
- Now, let go.
- Feel the relaxation in the muscles of the neck.

- Shrug the left shoulder to touch the earlobe.
- Feel the tightness in the muscles of the left shoulder.
- Now, let go.
- Feel the relaxation in the muscles of the left shoulder.

- Shrug the right shoulder to touch the earlobe.
- Feel the tightness in the muscles of the right shoulder.
- Now, let go.
- Feel the relaxation in the muscles of the right shoulder.

Step 5. **Relaxation of the Trunk (2 minutes)**

- Inhale deeply to tighten the chest muscles.
- Feel the tightness in the muscles of the chest.

Worksheet 3.2 Progressive Muscle Relaxation (cont'd)

- Now, let go.
- Feel the relaxation in the muscles of the chest.

- Exhale with force to tighten the abdominal muscles.
- Feel the tightness in the muscles of the abdomen.
- Now, let go.
- Feel the relaxation in the muscles of the abdomen.

Step 6. **Relaxation of the Whole Body (4 minutes)**

Give yourself the following autosuggestions (see Thoughts for Reflection 3.3).

- My feet are relaxed and healthy.
- My ankles are relaxed and healthy.
- My legs are relaxed and healthy.
- My knees are relaxed and healthy.
- My thighs are relaxed and healthy.
- My hips and pelvis are relaxed and healthy.
- My abdomen and parts within are relaxed and healthy.
- My chest and parts within are relaxed and healthy.
- My shoulders are relaxed and healthy.
- My arms are relaxed and healthy.
- My elbows are relaxed and healthy.
- My forearms are relaxed and healthy.
- My wrists are relaxed and healthy.
- My hands are relaxed and healthy.
- My neck is relaxed and healthy.
- My face is relaxed and healthy.
- My mind is relaxed and healthy.

FEEDBACK ON WORKSHEET 3.2

Progressive muscle relaxation is an excellent relaxation method with evidence to support its application as both prophylactic and therapeutic measures (Jacobson, 1938, 1977; McGuigan, 1993). The key to complete success lies in regular daily practice.

* * * * *

Thoughts for Reflection 3.3
Autosuggestion

Autosuggestion or talking with oneself is a powerful means to develop self-confidence and build healthy lifestyles. Dr. Emile Coué, a French psychotherapist, was the first to come up with the best-known phrase for autosuggestion—"Day by day in every way, I am getting better and better" (Patel, 1993). Reflect upon the following ideas for possible autosuggestions within the context of bringing relaxation in your life. After thinking through this list, you may wish to come up with a personal list of autosuggestions for yourself. These autosuggestions can be repeated to yourself during your free time or routinely during morning and evening or coupled with practice of other relaxation methods.

- I am happy, healthy, and relaxed.
- I am in harmony with my surroundings.
- I work efficiently and sufficiently.
- I enjoy complete peace of mind.
- My sleep is sound, refreshing, and relaxing.
- My relationship with self and others is cordial.
- I stay calm and relaxed even in potentially tense situations.
- All the organs and organ systems in my body are working and relaxing optimally.

* * * * *

Autogenic Training

Autogenic training (AT) owes its origin to the work of a German neurologist, Johannes Heinrich Schultz. He described it as a self-hypnotic procedure (Schultz, 1932). Autogenic therapy is a derivative of hypnosis and has been also described as "psychophysiological self-control therapy" (Pikoff, 1984).

Since this technique originated in Germany, it became and remains quite popular in European countries and Japan. This technique became known in North America when one of Schultz's followers, Wolfgang Luthe, a physician, emigrated to Canada and translated much of this work into English. There is ample evidence that it is a useful stress-reducing technique. It is also useful as a curative approach in dealing with anxiety and related disorders (Luthe, 1970). The term "autogenic" is derived from the Greek words *autos* meaning self, and *genos* meaning origin. Therefore, in this technique basically, the self-regulation and self-healing powers of the mind are channelized in a positive manner. The practitioner of autogenic training concentrates on his or her body sensations in a passive manner without directly or volitionally bringing about any change (Linden, 1993). The key sensations on which the mind is focused include those of *heaviness and warmth*. Focusing on these sensations provides the body with a feeling of relaxation because these sensations are normally associated with the relaxation process. With the help of Worksheet 3.3, you can now practice a slightly modified version of this technique that incorporates its key principles.

Worksheet 3.3
Autogenic Training

The following steps are a slight modification of the conventional autogenic training method developed by Schultz (1932). If practiced regularly, this method can reduce stress and provide effective relaxation.

Preparation

Choose a quiet and comfortable place. You may practice this method either in a sitting position or in a lying-down position. Choose a position in which you are comfortable. Close your eyes while practicing this technique. You may either repeat the suggestions in the following steps mentally or record them on a tape recorder and listen to the tape whenever you practice autogenic training.

Step 1. **Heaviness of the arms (2 minutes)**

- My right arm, forearm, and hand are getting heavy.
- I am feeling heaviness in my right arm, forearm, and hand.
- My left arm, forearm, and hand are getting heavy.
- I am feeling heaviness in my left arm, forearm, and hand.

Step 2. **Heaviness of the legs (2 minutes)**

- My right thigh, leg, and foot are getting heavy.
- I am feeling heaviness in my right thigh, leg, and foot.
- My left thigh, leg, and foot are getting heavy.
- I am feeling heaviness in my left thigh, leg, and foot.

Step 3. **Warmth in the arms (2 minutes)**

- My right arm, forearm, and hand are getting warm.
- I am feeling warmth in my right arm, forearm, and hand.
- My left arm, forearm, and hand are getting warm.
- I am feeling warmth in my left arm, forearm, and hand.

Step 4. **Warmth in the legs (2 minutes)**

- My right thigh, leg, and foot are getting warm.
- I am feeling warmth in my right thigh, leg, and foot.
- My left thigh, leg, and foot are getting warm.
- I am feeling warmth in my left thigh, leg, and foot.

Worksheet 3.3 Autogenic Training (cont'd)

***Step 5.* Strength of the heart (2 minutes)**

- My heartbeats are regular and steady.
- My heart is strong and healthy.
- I am feeling strength in my heart.

***Step 6.* Strength of breathing (2 minutes)**

- My breathing is regular and steady.
- My lungs are strong and healthy.
- My respiratory tract is clear and healthy.
- I am feeling strength in my lungs and respiratory tract.

***Step 7.* Strength of all visceral organs (2 minutes)**

- All my internal organs are healthy.
- I am feeling strength in all my internal organs.

***Step 8.* Coolness of the forehead (2 minutes)**

- My forehead is cool and relaxed.

***Step 9.* Finishing (1 minute)**

- My body and mind are completely relaxed and rested.

(Gradually open your eyes and get up.)

* * * * *

Visual Imagery

Visual imagery is mental visualization with the help of imagination. It is an important component of all relaxation procedures. It is somewhat akin to dreaming. It has been used both in the East and in the West. It is based on the principle that whatever we think and imagine has a profound impact on our body. The key emphasis of visual imagery lies in enhancing an individual's innate capacity to attain and maintain health (Miller & Lueth, 1978). This technique can be used to accomplish effective results in almost all spheres of life. For example, in the training of athletes and sportspersons, visual imagery is extensively utilized. Regular visual imagery training makes it possible for athletes to mentally visualize beforehand various situations (like performing in front of large crowds, winning an event, etc.) and techniques (like swinging a bat, shooting baskets, etc.). Regular practice of visual imagery has been shown to improve performance, especially in tournaments and competitions.

Within the context of relaxation, imagining relaxing scenes and images is a very useful way to bring about relaxation. Visual imagery can also be used to overcome barriers that hinder effective relaxation by mentally visualizing them beforehand. Worksheet 3.4 will help you to practice visual imagery for relaxation.

Thoughts for Reflection 3.3 provided you with some ideas for autosuggestions or self-talk that can enhance the benefits of relaxation.

Worksheet 3.4
Visual Imagery

Find a quiet and comfortable place. Leave aside all your other activities for at least half an hour. If possible, the place should not have any sources of possible distraction like telephones, small children playing, and so on. You may choose to lie down or sit.

- Close your eyes.
- Recollect the last time you were extremely happy. It may be that you were with someone; it may be that you had been somewhere; it may be that you got something. Whatever made you happy, mentally imagine that scene.
- Forget about everything else and just get engrossed in imagining that happy moment and scene.
- Remain with this feeling mentally for at least ten minutes.
- Now imagine any event that you may not have experienced but that you believe will make you happy.
- Mentally enjoy the feeling of being in that event.
- Be with this feeling for at least ten minutes.
- Now open your eyes and feel the relaxation and recharging of the system that has taken place.

* * * * *

Stress Management Principle 3

Make relaxation a part of your life.

Summary Points

- Relaxation is essential for normal functioning of all living beings. Relaxation techniques are the core of all stress management programs.
- The natural process of relaxation is sleep. Sleep conserves and restores energy.
- Sleep has two phases: rapid eye movement (REM) and non–rapid eye movement (non-REM). During the non-REM phase the mind reaches subtler frequencies as recorded on an electroencephalograph (EEG).
- Some of the techniques for relaxation are Yoga, meditation, Yogic breathing or *Pranayama,* biofeedback, progressive muscle relaxation (PMR), autogenic training (AT), and visual imagery.
- Yoga is a systematic application of the mind and body to achieve overall harmony and peace.
- Some systems of Yoga popular in the West include Transcendental Meditation (TM), *Kriya Yoga,* and *Simplified Kundalini Yoga.*
- Biofeedback utilizes instruments to provide awareness about bodily functions that may then be brought under voluntary control.
- Progressive Muscle Relaxation (PMR) was first described by Edmund Jacobson. It is an effective means of achieving relaxation.
- Autogenic Training was first described by J. H. Schultz and utilizes the self-regulation and self-healing processes of the mind to achieve relaxation.
- Visual Imagery or mental visualization with the help of imagination is an important component of all relaxation procedures.

References and Further Readings

Bernstein, D. A., & Borkovec, T. D. (1973). *Progressive relaxation training: A manual for the helping professions.* Champaign, IL: Research Press.

Bernstein, D. A., & Carlson, C. R. (1993). Progressive relaxation: Abbreviated methods. In P. M. Lehrer & R. L. Woolfolk (Eds.), *Principles and practice of stress management* (2nd ed.) (pp. 53–88). New York: Guilford Press.

Brown, B. (1974). *New mind, new body, biofeedback: New directions for the mind.* New York: Harper & Row.

Fuller, G. D. (1977). *Biofeedback: Methods and procedures in clinical practice.* San Francisco: Biofeedback Press.

Greenberg, J. S. (1999). *Comprehensive stress management* (6th ed). Boston: William C. Brown/McGraw-Hill.

Jacobson, E. (1938). *Progressive relaxation* (2nd ed.). Chicago: University of Chicago Press.

Jacobson, E. (1977). The origins and developments of progressive relaxation. *Journal of Behavior Therapy and Experimental Psychiatry, 8,* 119–123.

Kalat, J. W. (1988). *Biological psychology* (3rd ed.). New York: Wadsworth.

Karlins, M., & Andrews, L. W. (1972). *Biofeedback: Turning on the powers of your mind.* New York: J. B. Lippincott.

Kumar, C. S. C. (1993, August 29). What is TM? *The Week,* 10–15.

Linden, W. (1993). The autogenic training method of J. H. Schultz. In P. M. Lehrer & R. L. Woolfolk (Eds.), *Principles and practice of stress management* (2nd ed.) (pp. 53–88). New York: Guilford Press.

Luthe, W. (1970). *Autogenic therapy: Research and theory,* Vol. 4. New York: Grune & Stratton.

Maharishi, Y. V. (1986). *Karma yoga the holistic unity.* Madras, India: Vethathiri.

Maharishi, Y. V. (1987). *Simplified physical exercises.* Erode, India: Vethathiri.

Maharishi, Y. V. (1989). *Yoga for modern age.* Madras, India: Vethathiri.

McGuigan, F. J. (1993). Progressive relaxation: Origins, principles, and clinical applications. In P. M. Lehrer & R. L. Woolfolk (Eds.), *Principles and practice of stress management* (2nd ed.) (pp. 17–52). New York: Guilford Press.

Miller, E. E., & Lueth, D. (1978). *Self imagery: Creating your own good health.* Berkeley, CA: Celestial Arts.

Naranjo, C., & Ornstein, R. E. (1971). *On the psychology of meditation.* New York: Viking.

Patel C. (1993). Yoga based therapy. In P. M. Lehrer & R. L. Woolfolk (Eds.), *Principles and practice of stress management* (2nd ed.) (pp. 89–137). New York: Guilford Press.

Paul, G. L. (1966). *Insight versus desensitization in psychotherapy.* Stanford, CA: Stanford University Press.

Pikoff, H. (1984). A critical review of autogenic training in America. *Clinical Psychology Review, 4,* 619–639.

Schultz, J. H. (1932). *Das Autogene Training–Konzentrative Selbstentspannung.* [German]. Leipzig, Germany: Thieme.

Shapiro, C. M., & Flanigan, M. J. (1993). Function of sleep, *British Medical Journal, 306,* 383–385.

Singh, K. (1983). Hinduism. In *Religions of India.* New Delhi, India: Clarion Books.

Stoyva, J. M., & Budzynski, T. H. (1993). Biofeedback methods in the treatment of anxiety and stress disorders. In P. M. Lehrer & R. L. Woolfolk (Eds.), *Principles and practice of stress management* (2nd ed.) (pp. 263–300). New York: Guilford Press.

Vasu, R. B. S. C. (1915). *An introduction to the yoga philosophy.* Allahabad, India: Panini Office.

Wolpe, J. (1958). *Psychotherapy by reciprocal inhibition.* Stanford, CA: Stanford University Press.

Yogananda, P. (1946). *Autobiography of a yogi.* Los Angeles: Self-Realization Fellowship.

CHAPTER 4

Effective Communication

No Man Speaks . . .

No man speaks concerning another,
even suppose it be in his praise,
if he thinks he does not hear him,
exactly as he would,
if he thought he was within hearing.

—*Samuel Johnson*

What Is Communication?

We spend nearly 70 percent of our waking hours communicating—reading, writing, speaking, and listening (Robbins, 1998). If this communication becomes defective or faulty, it often leads to stress. Therefore, it is important for us to become effective communicators.

Before we proceed any further, let us first define the term "communication." One of the definitions that will come to mind will be "transfer of meaning." Is communication just "transfer of meaning"? Perhaps, it is more than just the transfer of meaning from one person to another. The important aspect of communication is the ability for the message to be understood—unless the meaning is understood, communication will remain incomplete and ineffective. These two aspects—transference and understanding of meaning—are extremely complex in their dimensions. Since we communicate very often, we seldom realize and appreciate the complexities involved.

Today, the English language has more than 600,000 words available. According to linguists, an average educated adult uses about 2000 of these words in daily conversation. But the problem is that out of these words, 500 of the words most frequently used have more than 14,000 dictionary definitions (Burke, Hall, & Hawley, 1986). And each one of us has his or her unique perspective in using and interpreting these words. More often than not this multiplicity leads to problematic communication. Furthermore, language is only a small tool that is used for communicating. A significant amount of communication occurs by means of our nonverbal gestures, tone of voice, and so on. Complicating the matter further, we have several models of communication available to us. In our contemporary world, communication by e-mail, Internet, and other technological advancements, while making the process faster, has also added several challenges (see Box 4.1).

Box 4.1 Computer Technology Advances: Newer Challenges for Stress Awareness

In present-day society, computer-aided communication is becoming a reality. Most of us have used e-mail for communicating to family, friends, relatives, and professional contacts. We may have also used the Internet for buying products, getting information, chatting, and several other considerations. Some of us may also have developed personal or professional home pages. All these are emerging forms of communication that add newer challenges to the process. Some of the challenges that this emerging technology is posing are as follows:

Novelty Effect: For the new user the process becomes emotionally stressful just because it is so new and learning has to take place from the beginning. Use of a computer as such may be new for many of us. To add the process of communication via computers becomes all the more stressful.

Less Time for Regular Communication: Many of us have become so accustomed to the new technology that we find less and less time for the traditional formal and informal means of communication. For many of us, this change creates a void in our normal day-to-day interactions and lessens our traditional social network. This reduction in conventional forms of networking also means reduction in conventional coping networks.

Speed of Communication: Technology is becoming faster, and we are able to communicate at a much faster speed. Therefore, there is less time for the thinking and proofreading that we are so used to in regular written communication. Oftentimes, this time pressure leads to miscommunication and creates stress for us and others.

Emerging and Fast-Changing Technology: In the computer world, technology is changing at a very fast pace. It implies that technology changes so fast that before we perfect something it becomes obsolete. This unprecedented fast pace is stressful.

Acronyms and Abbreviations: People who are using more and more computer-aided communication are finding and learning so many new words, use of language in a different way, abbreviations, acronyms, and use of symbols to depict mood and feelings. For example, the acronym "lol" is used to convey the feeling "laughing out loud." Use of such newer forms can add stress for the neophyte.

Junk Mail and Spamming: Sometimes computer-aided communication is being used by some people to vent their stress in the form of sending a lot of irrelevant junk mail to others (spamming). Besides stressing the network—it is stressful for all humans involved too!

While it may indeed be true that change is for the good and so are technological advancements—a little reflection on what these technological advancements and changes mean for us and our stress levels may give us a better insight into improving upon our communication and reducing the stress levels in our lives.

* * * * *

The Communication Process

Communication was first described as a process by Berlo (1960). This model, known as the SMCR Model (Sender, Message, Channel, Receiver), is one of the most popular (Figure 4.1). The message to be conveyed passes between the sender (the source) and the receiver. The message is converted to a symbolic form (encoded) and is passed by way of some channel (medium) to the receiver who retranslates (decodes) the message initiated by the sender. In this way transference of meaning from one person to another results.

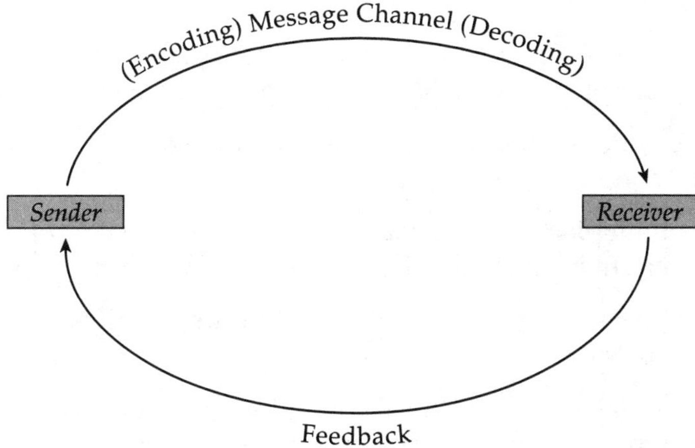

Figure 4.1 Berlo's SMCR Model of Communication

Let us try to understand what goes into each of these components. The *sender* initiates communication by *encoding* or converting a communication message to symbolic form. This process is influenced by the following factors:

- Knowledge or information about the message—the factual components that may be correct or incorrect
- Skills like writing, speaking, etc.—the ability level of the sender to articulate the message
- Beliefs that are convictions that a phenomenon or object is true or real (Rokeach, 1970)—the impressions about the world
- Attitudes that are constant feelings directed toward an object (person, situation, or idea) and have an evaluative dimension (Green & Kreuter, 1991; Mucchielli, 1970)—beliefs with an evaluative component
- Values or cultural intergenerational perspectives (Rokeach, 1970)—enduring set of attitudes and beliefs that a mode of conduct is personally or socially preferable

The *message* is the actual physical product from the sender encoding it. For example, when we speak, the speech is the message; when we write, the writing is the message; when we gesture, the body movements are the message; and so on.

The medium through which a communication message travels is the *channel.* Myers and Nance (1991) in *The Upset Book* have identified seven channels of communication, namely:

1. Language—this is the "what" part of the message, the actual content or gist of the matter being conveyed.
2. Manner—this is how we express the message or say it vocally. The way in which a message is conveyed sometimes assumes greater importance than even the gist of what is said.
3. Body language—this is how we express the message visually through our body movements. Use of gestures and actions adds flavor to the message.
4. Feelings or emotions—these are often inseparable from the communication process and get easily and automatically conveyed.
5. Symbolic communication—for example, dress, hairstyle, appearance, and so on are also important components that get consciously or unconsciously noticed.
6. Territory—this is personal space that includes both physiological and psychological dimensions.
7. Behavior—this includes intentional and not so intentional actions. The frequency, intensity, and duration of these actions can be documented.

The *receiver* is the object to whom the message is directed. But before the message can be received, the symbols in it must be translated into a form that can be deciphered. This is the *decoding* and is influenced by similar factors as discussed in encoding earlier. The final link in the communication process is a *feedback loop,* which puts the message back into the system as a check against misunderstandings. All of these seven components are subject to possible distortion and can thereby contribute to the causes of stress.

You should now assess your ability to communicate through Worksheet 4.1. Worksheet 4.2 will help you identify your communication process in various situations and will provide feedback on ways to improve communication.

Worksheet 4.1
Communication Assessment

This worksheet is a self-assessment tool that will enhance your awareness of various attributes of effective communication and has no right or wrong answers. It can also be used for gathering feedback from others about you as a communicator. So you can ask your spouse, a family member, friend, colleague, or someone who knows you to fill out this worksheet for you.

How would you rate yourself (or the person whom you are assessing) on the following items?

Excellent, 5; very good, 4; satisfactory, 3; poor, 2; very poor, 1:

While communicating . . .	**Rating Scale**				
1. I am concise and to the point.	5	4	3	2	1
2. I express myself clearly.	5	4	3	2	1
3. I modulate the tone of my voice to convey precise meaning.	5	4	3	2	1
4. I use appropriate body gestures and facial expressions.	5	4	3	2	1
5. I am forceful and definite rather than hesitant and apologetic.	5	4	3	2	1
6. I summarize the key points.	5	4	3	2	1
7. I do not talk in roundabout ways.	5	4	3	2	1
8. I am specific and give examples to make my points clear.	5	4	3	2	1
9. I let others know in unambiguous terms when I do not follow them.	5	4	3	2	1
10. I often ask others if they have followed me.	5	4	3	2	1

Worksheet 4.1 Communication Assessment (cont'd)

11. I help others participate in the discussion.	5	4	3	2	1
12. I listen actively.	5	4	3	2	1
13. I keep my feelings under check.	5	4	3	2	1
14. I do not react to the feelings of others.	5	4	3	2	1
15. I listen to understand rather than prepare for the next remark.	5	4	3	2	1
16. I avoid using jargon and use simple language.	5	4	3	2	1
17. I give equal respect to others as communicators.	5	4	3	2	1
18. I try to see the other person's point of view.	5	4	3	2	1
19. I do not divert myself while communicating.	5	4	3	2	1
20. I am able to withstand silence.	5	4	3	2	1

FEEDBACK ON WORKSHEET 4.1

Having rated yourself and also having elicited feedback from others, you will now be quite clear about your strengths and limitations. Try to build further on your strengths (categories in which you have rated excellent and very good). Also try to overcome your limitations (categories in which you have rated yourself or have been rated as satisfactory, poor, or very poor).

* * * * *

Worksheet 4.2
Communication in Various Situations

This worksheet provides you with certain situations. Circle the answer that best describes what you would do in each situation.

1. I have an important appointment in the next one-half hour and my best friend arrives. I would . . .

   a. ask my spouse to handle the situation and leave from the back door.
   b. exchange pleasantries and excuse myself politely.
   c. cancel the appointment.
   d. hurriedly leave.

2. I need to imagine myself to be working in a middle management position. The head of the organization invites me for lunch. When I return, I sense that my department head is curious. I would . . .

   a. ignore him or her.
   b. give a detailed description.
   c. mention the meeting casually—as though nothing has happened.
   d. fabricate a story.

3. My boyfriend (or girlfriend) is not able to keep a date with me. I would . . .

   a. act as if nothing has happened.
   b. ask him or her the reasons.
   c. wait for his or her explanations.
   d. walk out on him or her.

4. My spouse tells me a juicy story about the neighbor's daughter that he or she has heard from somewhere. I would say . . .

   a. "I don't want to hear any of this."
   b. "I am not interested."
   c. "What happened next?"
   d. "How does it concern us?"

5. I have to stay late at the office completing pending work. I return home and am tired. My spouse inquires the reason for my coming in late. I would . . .

   a. tell my spouse to mind his or her own business.
   b. explain the reason clearly.
   c. ignore him or her.
   d. change the topic of conversation.

Worksheet 4.2 Communication in Various Situations (cont'd)

6. My supervisor, in a staff meeting, makes an inaccurate statement. I would . . .

   a. correct my supervisor on the spot.
   b. correct my supervisor later away from the meeting.
   c. ask a clarifying question at the meeting and discuss the matter later.
   d. tell other staff members how foolish my supervisor is.

7. I am at a party, and someone introduces me to a person of different ethnic orientation. After initiating conversation, I am unable to understand the other person. I would . . .

   a. politely excuse myself.
   b. ask the person for repeated clarifications.
   c. nod in agreement.
   d. form an opinion about his/her poor communication skills.

8. A friend calls me on the phone and invites me to a sports event. I have made other plans with another person but would very much like to go. I would . . .

   a. call my other friend and cancel the appointment so I can go to the sports event.
   b. ask my friend if the other person can come along to the sports event.
   c. persuade my friend to cancel going to the sports event and join me.
   d. cancel both engagements and stay at home.

9. I enter a meeting and find that all the members have burst into laughter. I would . . .

   a. assume that they are laughing at me and leave the meeting.
   b. assume that they are laughing at me and speak against their inappropriate behavior.
   c. laugh with them and later ask the reason for laughing.
   d. sit quietly and ask nothing.

10. I give my teenage son or daughter a specific time to be home. He or she openly defies my directive by coming home very late. I would . . .

    a. reprimand him or her and decide not to talk about it again.
    b. discuss the matter openly the next day.
    c. blame my spouse for spoiling the teenager.
    d. call up the other parents and complain.

FEEDBACK ON WORKSHEET 4.2

The most appropriate responses that would help prevent undue stress from occurring in your life because of improper communication are as follows:

1. b This response would prevent any miscommunication and misunderstanding to occur.
2. b You owe your loyalty to your immediate supervisor. If you fabricate or ignore or do not tell enough, you will sow the seeds of mistrust and create stress later.
3. b An open discussion would help you understand his or her problem and avoid undue stress.
4. d You need to avoid gossip that floats around unless it concerns you and then try to find the facts. In this way miscommunication and associated problems leading to stress can be avoided.
5. b This response would prevent any miscommunication and misunderstanding from occurring.
6. c Asking a clarification question at the time of the discussion will help your supervisor to correct himself or herself, if he or she has made the statement out of oversight. If not, discussion at a later time will help clarify your point of view without embarrassing your supervisor.
7. b Repeated clarifications will help you gain an understanding of what the other person is trying to communicate and lessen stress for both of you.
8. b Accomplishing your goals without hurting the feelings of others is a part of assertiveness and effective communication. Being up front about your position will help to reduce stress.
9. c Laughing with people, even if you are being laughed at, will reduce undue discomfort to you. Soliciting clarification later on will help you understand the actual reason.
10. b An open discussion about the matter will help both of you to clarify your viewpoints and reach mutual understanding to reduce family stress.

This worksheet should help you appreciate the importance of straightforwardness and assertiveness in your communication with others in order to reduce stress.

* * * * *

Assertiveness

Another important aspect of communication is the ability to say no, if you want to say no, without feeling guilty. This is known as being assertive. Assertiveness has been defined as "expressing personal rights and feelings" (Lazarus, 1966; Wolpe, 1958). In another way it can be defined as expressing oneself, satisfying one's personal needs, feeling good about this, and not hurting others in the process (Greenberg, 1999). Worksheet 4.3, Assessing Assertive Behavior, will help you to gain insight into passive, assertive, and aggressive behaviors when communicating with others.

Research shows that nearly everybody can be assertive in some situations, whereas in others the same person will be ineffectual. The goal therefore is to increase the number and variety of situations in which assertive behavior is possible. This decreases the events in which a passive behavior or a hostile blowup will occur.

Assertiveness is not the same as aggressiveness. One can differentiate between the two by asking three simple questions:

1. Am I violating someone else's rights?
2. Do others react to me by getting angry or upset?
3. Do I intend to be malicious or do I intend to be fair to all concerned?

Aggressiveness means seeking to dominate or to get your own way at the expense of others. This tendency should be curbed as far as possible and replaced with assertiveness. Practice to be more assertive as shown in Worksheet 4.4.

Thoughts for Reflection 4.1
A Bill of Assertive Rights

1. You have the right to judge your own behavior, thoughts, and emotions, and to take responsibility for their initiation and consequences upon yourself.
2. You have the right to offer no reasons or excuses for your behavior.
3. You have the right to judge if you are responsible for finding solutions to other people's problems.
4. You have the right to change your mind.
5. You have the right to make mistakes—and be responsible for them.
6. You have the right to say, " I don't know."
7. You have the right to be independent of the goodwill of others before coping with them.
8. You have the right to be illogical in making decisions.
9. You have the right to say, "I don't understand."
10. You have the right to say, "I don't care."

Note: From *When I say no, I feel guilty* by Manuel J. Smith. Copyright © 1975 by Manuel J. Smith. Used by permission of Doubleday, a division of Bantam Doubleday Dell Publishing Group, Inc.

* * * * *

Worksheet 4.3
Assessing Assertive Behavior

To determine your general pattern of behavior, indicate how characteristic or descriptive of you each of the following statements is by using the code that follows:

+3 = very characteristic of me, extremely descriptive
+2 = rather characteristic of me, quite descriptive
+1 = somewhat characteristic of me, slightly descriptive
–1 = somewhat uncharacteristic of me, slightly nondescriptive
–2 = rather uncharacteristic of me, quite nondescriptive
–3 = very uncharacteristic of me, extremely nondescriptive

____ 1. Most people seem to be more aggressive and assertive than I am.

____ 2. I have hesitated to make or accept dates because of "shyness."

____ 3. When the food served at a restaurant is not done to my satisfaction, I complain about it to the waiter or waitress.

____ 4. I am careful to avoid hurting other people's feelings, even when I feel that I have been injured.

____ 5. If a salesperson has gone to considerable trouble to show me merchandise that is not quite suitable, I have a difficult time in saying no.

____ 6. When I am asked to do something, I insist upon knowing why.

____ 7. There are times when I look for a good, vigorous argument.

____ 8. I strive to get ahead as well as most people in my position.

____ 9. To be honest, people often take advantage of me.

____ 10. I enjoy starting conversations with new acquaintances and strangers.

____ 11. I often don't know what to say to attractive persons of the opposite sex.

____ 12. I will hesitate to make phone calls to business establishments and institutions.

____ 13. I would rather apply for a job or for admission to a college by writing letters than by going through with personal interviews.

____ 14. I find it embarrassing to return merchandise.

Worksheet 4.3 Assessing Assertive Behavior (cont'd)

____ 15. If a close and respected relative were annoying me, I would smother my feeling rather than express my annoyance.

____ 16. I have avoided asking questions for fear of sounding stupid.

____ 17. During an argument I am sometimes afraid that I will get so upset that I will shake all over.

____ 18. If a famed and respected lecturer makes a statement that I think is incorrect, I will have the audience hear my point of view.

____ 19. I avoid arguing over prices with clerks and sales people.

____ 20. When I have done something important or worthwhile, I manage to let others know about it.

____ 21. I am open and frank about my feelings.

____ 22. If someone has been spreading false and bad stories about me, I see him or her as soon as possible to "have a talk" about it.

____ 23. I often have a hard time saying no.

____ 24. I tend to bottle up my emotions rather than make a scene.

____ 25. I complain about poor service in a restaurant and elsewhere.

____ 26. When I am given a compliment, I sometimes just don't know what to say.

____ 27. If a couple near me in a theater or at a lecture were conversing rather loudly, I would ask them to be quiet or to take their conversation elsewhere.

____ 28. Anyone attempting to push ahead of me in a line is in for a good battle.

____ 29. I am quick to express an opinion.

____ 30. There are times when I just can't say anything.

Note: From "A 30 item schedule for assessing assertive behavior" by S. A. Rathus, 1973, *Behavior Therapy 4*, 398–406. Copyright 1973 by Academic Press. Reprinted by permission.

FEEDBACK ON WORKSHEET 4.3

To score this scale, first change (reverse) the signs (+ or –) for your scores on items 1, 2, 4, 5, 9, 11, 12, 13, 14, 15, 16, 17, 19, 23, 24, 26, and 30. Now total the plus (+) items, total the minus (–) items, and subtract the minus total from the plus total to obtain your score. This score can range from –90 through 0 to +90. The higher the score (closer to 90), the more assertively you usually behave. The lower the score (closer to –90), the more nonassertive is your typical behavior. This particular scale does not measure aggressiveness.

* * * * *

Worksheet 4.4
Five Steps to Becoming Assertive

The following is a step-by-step process to become more assertive. Find a quiet place to work on this worksheet, and proceed as directed.

Step 1. Identification of an Environmental Situation

You need to identify an environmental situation on which you want feedback. It may be your work situation, or it may be your personal life or something else. Write it down in the following space:

____

____

Step 2. Behavior Style Classification

Identify and encircle your style of interpersonal behavior as

- *Passive:* avoids problems, allows manipulation by others, gives up one's rights, and lacks self-confidence. This type of behavior is stress producing.
- *Assertive:* faces problems, gains respect from others by letting them know one's opinions, claims rights, and has self-confidence. This type of behavior is least stress producing.
- *Aggressive:* attacks the other person, takes advantage of people, disregards the rights of others, and is often hostile. This type of behavior is most stress producing.

Reasons:

____

____

Step 3. Person Identification

All situations involve some persons. Identify the persons with whom you would like to be more assertive. List them here:

____

____

Worksheet 4.4 Five Steps to Becoming Assertive (cont'd)

Step 4. **Script Writing**

Write a script for changing your actions and reactions in order to become more assertive with these people.

a. Identify your rights and feelings—define your goal.

____

____

____

____

____

____

b. Describe your feelings by using "I" statements. For example, "I like to . . . ," "I shall . . ."

____

____

____

____

____

____

Step 5. **Discussion Session**

Have a discussion with the person with whom you would like to be more assertive using the following checklist:

- Arrange a time and place for discussion.
- Concisely *define* the problem.
- *Describe* your feelings in "I" messages.

Worksheet 4.4 Five Steps to Becoming Assertive (cont'd)

- Make your *request* in a brief sentence or two.
- *Reinforce* the other person's thinking by stating positive consequences of cooperation and if necessary negative consequences for failure to cooperate.
- Use assertive *body language* like direct eye contact, erect body posture, clarity of speech.
- Avoid manipulation.
- Be willing to compromise if it is essential.

* * * * *

Worksheets 4.3 and 4.4 have provided you with an insight as to whether or not you are assertive. Some characteristics of an assertive person include

- Direct eye contact
- Appropriate use of hand movements
- Firm posture
- Steady utilization of voice
- Use of "I" statements
- Speech meanings conveyed in short sentences
- Feedback pauses

A person exhibiting assertiveness always uses direct eye contact by looking the other person in the eye while communicating. An assertive person utilizes appropriate hand movements while communicating, being careful not to cause discomfort or invade the other person's space. An assertive person engages in a firm posture, not too stiff, yet not too relaxed, which maintains an appropriate distance in which both parties are comfortable. An assertive person uses a steady, consistent voice, keeping emotion to a minimum. One of the key characteristics of an assertive person is the use of "I" statements when speaking, which demonstrates to others that an assertive person owns his or her behavior and is responsible for any consequence thereof. An assertive person uses short sentences expressing clarity and brevity in thought. Finally, an assertive person often pauses to obtain feedback from others, which is vital for effective communication to take place. Thoughts for Reflection 4.2 provides some ideas for becoming assertive, and Thoughts for Reflection 4.3 describes nine types of assertive responses.

Thoughts for Reflection 4.2
Assertive Communication Techniques

- *Broken Record.* A systematic communication skill in which one is persistent and keeps saying what one wants over and over again without getting angry, irritated, or loud. By practicing to speak like a broken record, we learn to be persistent, to stick to the point of discussion, and to continue to say what we want. This technique helps us to ignore all side issues brought up by the other party.
- *Workable Compromise.* A technique to utilize with an equally assertive person to work out a compromise. A workable compromise is one in which our self-respect is not in question.
- *Free Information.* A listening skill in which we evaluate and then follow up on the free information that people offer about themselves. It accomplishes two things. It makes it easier for us to converse comfortably with people, and it is assertively prompting to others to speak easily and freely with us.
- *Self-Disclosure.* Assertively disclosing information about ourselves. How we think, feel, and react to the other person's free information—permits social communication to flow both ways. It goes hand in hand with free information because in order to elicit more information, we must be willing for self-disclosure.
- *Fogging.* A technique to assertively cope with manipulative criticism, in which we do not deny any of the criticism, we do not get defensive, and we do not attack with criticism of our own. We send up a fog bank. It is persistent. It cannot be clearly seen through. It offers no resistance to penetration. It does not fight back and has no hard striking surfaces. Fogging permits us to cope by offering no resistance or hard psychological striking surfaces to critical statements thrown at us.
- *Negative Assertion.* A technique in which we cope with criticism or with our own errors and faults by openly acknowledging them. This technique is to be used only in social conflicts and not physical or legal ones.
- *Negative Inquiry.* An assertive, nondefensive response that is noncritical of the other person and prompts that person to make further critical statements to examine his or her own structure of right and wrong which he or she is using in certain situations, e.g., "I don't understand. What makes you think educators are stupid?"

Note: From *Stress stoppers: Managing stress effectively* (p. 25) by P. R. Kovacek, 1981, Detroit: Henry Ford Hospital. Material under public domain.

* * * * *

Thoughts for Reflection 4.3
Nine Types of Assertive Responses

1. *Assertive Talk:* Do not let others take advantage of you. Expect to be treated with fairness and justice. Example: "I was here first," "Please turn down the radio," "I've been waiting here for half an hour," and "This steak is well-done and I ordered it medium-rare."

2. *Feeling Talk:* Express your likes and dislikes spontaneously. Be open and frank about your feelings. Do not bottle up emotions, but don't let emotions control you. Examples: "What a marvelous shirt!" "How great you look!" "I hate this cold," "I'm tired as hell," "Since you ask, I do prefer you in another type of outfit."

3. *Greeting Talk:* Be outgoing and friendly with people whom you would like to know better. Do not avoid people because of shyness, because you do not know what to say. Smile brightly at people. Look and sound pleased to see them. Examples: "Hi, how are you?" "Hello, I haven't seen you in months," "What are you doing with yourself these days?" "How do you like working at ____________________ ?" "Taking any good courses?" "What's been happening with so and so?"

4. *Disagreeing Passively and Actively:* When you disagree with someone, do not feign agreement for the sake of "keeping the peace" by smiling, nodding, or paying close attention. Change the topic. Look away. Disagree actively when you are sure of your ground. Use fogging with manipulative criticizers.

5. *Asking Why:* When you are asked to do something that does not sound reasonable or enjoyable by a person in power or authority, ask why you should do it. You are an adult and should not accept authority alone. Ask for reasonable explanations from teachers, relatives, and other authority figures. Have it understood that you will live up to voluntary commitments and be open to reasonable suggestions, but that you cannot comply with unreasonable orders.

6. *Talking about Oneself:* When you have done something worthwhile or interesting, let others know about it. Let people know how you feel about things. Relate *your* experiences. Do not monopolize conversations, but do not be afraid to bring them around to yourself when it is appropriate.

7. *Agreeing with Compliments:* Do not depreciate yourself or become flustered when someone compliments you with sincerity. At the very least, offer an equally sincere "Thank you." Or reward the complimenter by saying, "That's an awfully nice thing to say. I appreciate it."

Thoughts for Reflection 4.3 Nine Types of Assertive Responses (cont'd)

8. *Avoid Trying Justification of Opinions:* Be reasonable in discussions, but when someone goes out of his/her way to dominate a social interaction by taking issue with any comments you offer, use a technique like "broken record."

9. *Looking People in the Eye:* Do not avoid the gaze of others. When you argue, express an opinion, or greet a person, look him or her directly in the eye.

Note: Adapted from *Behavior research & therapy. II,* S. A. Rathus, "Instigation of assertive behavior through video tape mediated assertive models and directed practice," pp. 57–65. Copyright © 1973 with kind permission from Elsevier Science Ltd., The Boulevard, Langford Lane, Kidlington, OX5 1GB, UK.

* * * * *

Behavioral Styles

Now that we have practiced assertiveness, let us focus our attention on another important aspect of communication, that is, on how we behave. All of us have developed certain behavioral patterns—distinct ways of thinking, feeling, and acting. The central core of these patterns tends to remain stable because it reflects our individual identities. However, the demands of the world around us (namely, personal, family, school, and work) often require different responses that evolve into a consistent behavioral style (Carlson Learning Company, 1994). One of the tools to explain behavioral styles is the Personal Profile System® developed by Carlson Learning Company of Minneapolis, Minnesota. This profile presents a plan to help us understand ourselves and others in our social or work environment.

This Personal Profile System is a self-administered, self-development instrument. The profile was originally developed by Dr. John Geier based upon extensive study of our behavioral tendencies and subsequently refined by Dr. Michael O'Connor (Carlson Learning Company, 1994). The Personal Profile also utilizes the work of William Moulton Marston. He had theorized that human behavior could be studied on a two-axis model according to a person's actions in a favorable or an antagonistic environment (Marston, 1979).

The focus of this instrument is to understand oneself so that one can understand others and place oneself in an environment that is conducive to one's success (Kaufman & O'Connor, 1992). This instrument measures four dimensions of behavioral responses (DiSC, Carlson Learning Company, 1994):

- Dominance (D): emphasis is on shaping the environment by overcoming opposition to accomplish results.
- Influence (i): emphasis is on shaping the environment by influencing or persuading others.
- Steadiness (S): emphasis is on cooperation with others to carry out the task.
- Conscientiousness (C): emphasis is on cautious, tentative response designed to reduce antagonistic factors in an unfavorable environment.

The behavioral dimensions can be divided into two categories—process or product orientation. Persons with predominantly *Dominance* or *Influence* tendencies are process oriented. They want to shape the environment according to their particular view. These are individuals who continually test and push the limits set by the group or organization. Those people with the *Steadiness* and *Conscientiousness* tendencies are product oriented. They focus on the how and the why. These people may at times need encouragement to reset limits.

For example, people with *Dominance tendencies* have the results they want well in mind. Their messages are designed to stimulate and prod others to untested action. They are attentive to communication that will speed up the action. Questions about the "correct" action are shrugged away. These individuals feel they can change the course of action (Performax Systems International, 1986).

People with *Influence tendencies* also want to shape and mold events and have an active voice. Their messages are designed to stimulate and prod others to action by working with and through people. They are interested in people and like to make people feel good about themselves. They are particularly attentive to the personal needs of others and search for ways in which to meet these needs. Messages about how to actually accomplish a task are often deemed unimportant; these stimuli are at the far range of their attention span.

Persons with *Steadiness tendencies* are interested in how and when—a product orientation. They send messages that reflect their interest in maintaining a stability within themselves and the situation—between the old and the new. Messages that urge action before knowing how to do things fall on deaf ears.

Those individuals with the *Conscientiousness (to their own standards) tendencies* reflect their product orientation when they send messages that ask the reasons for the change. "Why?" is a favorite question. They have concern for doing it "accurately." They are receptive to messages that reassure them they are doing it correctly. Messages that ignore this need tend to go unheeded.

How the Personal Profile Contributes to Stress Reduction

The Personal Profile System provides considerable information about the way people respond to stress. This information can be effectively utilized to understand and help reduce stress. As we have seen earlier, in Chapters 1 and 2 the stress response consists of two components: "fight" or "flight." Hans Selye (1956) refined this concept into four distinct responses that correspond to our four primary behavioral tendencies as outlined in the following list:

- *Fight*—The high "D" will tend to use the fight response. They will attempt to destroy the impact of the stress or eliminate its cause. The fighting may be verbal or physical.
- *Flight*—The high "i" will tend to use the flight response. They will attempt to flee from the situation. If physical flight is not possible, they will attempt to flee emotionally by changing the subject or ignoring the issue. If the stress continues, they may become emotionally abusive.
- *Tolerate*—The high "S" will tend to use the tolerate response, which is really a subtle form of flight. They will not attempt to flight or flee; however, they will tend to shut down. They will remain in the situation with apparent calmness; however, they may become dysfunctional, not knowing what to do.
- *Avoid*—The high "C" will tend to use the avoid response, which is a subtle form of fight. They will not attempt to fight or flee; however, they will tend to withdraw in order to avoid conflict. They may, in fact, use the time as an opportunity to carefully plan their next move.

According to Kaufman and O'Connor (1992), if the level of stress becomes even more severe, the individuals will tend to move step by step through the stress responses associated with behavioral styles more directive than their own. That is, a "high i" will first move from the flight response to the tolerate response characteristic of the "high S."

This individual will then move from the "tolerate" response to the "avoid" response to the "fight" response characteristic of the "high D." A "high S" individual will move through the "avoid" response to the "fight" response. A "high C" individual will move to the "fight" response. The "fight" response is the ultimate survival-level response. We will all resort to that behavior if the level of stress is high enough.

For further information and training on the Personal Profile System, one may contact J.A.R. and Associates, Management, Training, & Health Consultants, 407 West Eighth Street, Suite 333, Mankato, MN, 56001; telephone (507) 345–8822, fax (507) 345–8534, e-mail:< jar@ic.mankato.mn.us>.

Note: Information on behavioral styles is adapted from the widely used DiSC™ Dimensions of Behavior Model and the Personal Profile System.® © Copyright 1994, Carlson Learning Company.

Stress Management Principle 4

Think first before passing judgment.

Summary Points

- We spend approximately two-thirds of our waking hours in communicating.
- Faulty communication is at the root of most stress.
- A popular model of communication described by Berlo is known as the SMCR (Sender, Message, Channel, Receiver) Model.
- An important aspect of communication is assertiveness or the ability to say no without feeling guilty.
- Being assertive produces the least amount of stress, whereas being passive or aggressive is more stressful.
- Assertiveness is an acquired quality, and all of us can learn to be assertive.
- Some of the techniques for becoming assertive include sounding like a broken record, compromising, providing free information, self-disclosure, fogging, negative assertion, and negative inquiry.
- How we behave impacts upon how effectively we communicate.
- The Personal Profile System is a tool to assess our behavioral styles. The Profile describes four responses: Dominance (D), Influence (i), Steadiness (S), and Conscientiousness (C).

References and Further Readings

Allessandra, T., O'Connor, M. J., & Allessandra, J. (1990). *People smart: Powerful techniques for turning every encounter into a mutual win.* La Jolla, CA: Keynote.

Berlo, D. K. (1960). *The process of communication.* New York: Holt, Rinehart and Winston.

Bower, S. A., & Bower, G. H. (1976). *Asserting yourself.* Reading, MA: Addison-Wesley.

Burke, C. R., Hall, D. R., & Hawley, D. (1986). *Living with stress.* Clackamas, OR: Wellsource.

Carlson Learning Company. (1994). *The Personal Profile System.* Minneapolis: Carlson Learning Company.

Davis, M. , Eshelman, E. R., & McKay, M. (1982). *The relaxation and stress reduction workbook* (2nd ed.). Oakland, CA: New Harbinger.

Green, L. W., & Kreuter, M. W. (1991). *Health promotion planning: An educational and environmental approach* (2nd ed.). Mountain View, CA: Mayfield.

Greenberg, J. S. (1999). *Comprehensive stress management* (6th ed.). Boston: William C. Brown/McGraw-Hill.

Kaufman, D., & O'Connor, M. J. (1992). *Basic questions and answer guide for needs motivated behavior.* Minneapolis: Carlson Marketing Group.

Kovacek, P. R. (1981). Stress stoppers: Managing stress effectively. Detroit: Henry Ford Hospital.

Lazarus, A. A. (1966). Behaviour rehearsal vs. nondirective therapy vs. advice in effecting behaviour change. *Behaviour Research and Therapy, 4,* 209–212.

Marston, W. M. (1979). *Emotions of normal people.* Minneapolis: Personal Press.

Mucchielli, R. (1970). *Introduction to structural psychology.* New York: Funk & Wagnalls.

Myers, P., & Nance, D. (1991). *The upset book* (2nd ed.). Wichita, KS: Mac Press.

O'Connor, M. J., & Merwin, S. J. (1992). *The mysteries of motivation: Why people do the things they do.* Minneapolis: Carlson Learning Company.

Performax Systems International. (1986). *The personal profile system manual and behavioral patterns master guide.* Minneapolis: Carlson Learning Company.

Rathus, S. A. (1973). A 30 item schedule for assessing assertive behavior. *Behavior Therapy, 4,* 398–406.

Robbins, S. P. (1998). *Organizational behavior: Concepts, controversies, and applications* (8th ed.). Paramus, NJ: Prentice Hall.

Rokeach, M. (1970). *Beliefs, attitudes and values.* San Francisco: Jossey Bass.

Selye, H. (1956). *The stress of life.* New York: McGraw-Hill.

Smith, M. J. (1975). *When I say no, I feel guilty.* New York: Bantam Books.

Wolpe, J. (1958). *Psychotherapy by reciprocal inhibition.* Stanford, CA: Stanford University Press.

Yogananda, P. (1946). *Autobiography of a yogi.* Los Angeles: Self-Realization Fellowship.

CHAPTER 5

Managing Anger and Resolving Conflicts

A Poison Tree

I was angry with my friend
I told my wrath, my wrath did end.
I was angry with my foe:
I told it not, my wrath did grow.

—*William Blake*

What Is Anger?

Anger is an emotion that, if not managed, neutralized, or controlled, can result in great suffering for oneself, as well as for others. Uncontrolled anger results in release of various hormones and neurotransmitters. As a consequence, blood pressure rises, cardiac muscles contract, and gastric secretions increase. Eventually the by-products produced do not get used in the system and accumulate causing harm to the body. This buildup can manifest itself in the form of various illnesses such as hypertension, peptic ulcer, stroke, and others. Psychologically, uncontrolled anger "poisons the mind" and makes us perform many actions that we may regret later. At the societal level anger is at the root of many wars, terrorist activities, riots, looting, arson, domestic abuse, road rage, workplace violence, divorce, and so on. Therefore, the anger that originates within the mind gradually engulfs the body and the family and eventually has devastating effects on society. However, some anger within limits and with *full awareness* is beneficial too because it protects the human organism. The key, however, is to have *balance* with anger. In this chapter we will discuss how to attain this balance.

Most of us tend to "blow up" at the slightest provocation. Later we regret our behavior when it is usually too late. According to Smith (1993), when considering anger, it is useful to begin by making some distinctions. Anger that results in aggression is destructive *behavior*. However, anger is essentially an internal *feeling*. While it is often appropriate to monitor and control aggressive behavior, feelings cannot always be controlled. It is important to realize that the feeling of anger can serve as a useful warning sign that we may be about to engage in aggressive or self-destructive behavior. Therefore, it is important to manage one's anger and attain a state of balance.

We have a number of diagnostic tests available for various medical disorders, but unfortunately no standard test is available for diagnosing anger. Moreover, a number of questions about anger continue to perplex and challenge us. For example, do we consider whether or not angry people are sick? Does getting angry make us feel better? If we let our anger out, what are the consequences? If we hold our anger in, what are the consequences?

Managing the Anger Within

Most psychologists agree that if we become angry, we must feel that anger. There is no point in denying, hiding, repressing, or suppressing that anger. This overt feeling is a natural process. We can appreciate that a newborn infant expresses these emotions of anger and rage by crying out at the time of birth. Throughout all ages or periods of development, many humans confront almost daily their own feelings of anger and those of other people with whom they come in contact. It is generally accepted today that we need our anger to protect us from a hostile and aggressive world.

Unfortunately, we generally tend to do one of the following when dealing with anger within: (1) feel the anger, but sit on it, deny it, and repress it; or (2) feel the anger and freely express it. Denial and repression of our anger does not get us anywhere, and "uncontrolled rage" leads to far more harm.

A well-known model to manage anger is based upon the concepts of Rational Emotive Therapy (RET) developed by Albert Ellis (1975, 1977). He proposed the *hydraulic theory,* which states that anger and other emotions have a tendency to increase in intensity, to expand under pressure like steam in a kettle, so that if we "squelch" our emotions, if we do not give free vent to them, we run the risk of doing some real harm to ourselves. Real physical harm such as stomach ulcers, high blood pressure, or other ailments, including severe psychosomatic reactions, may ensue.

Conversely, if we let ourselves feel authentically angry (*free expression*) and let others know about our feelings, we may frequently encounter problems of quite another nature. People will receive our free expression of anger in most instances as an outwardly aggressive or hostile action, and will probably close themselves off from us and defensively respond to us with further hostility. Some therapists in the field have attempted to solve the problem with still another alternative, which they call *creative aggression* (or *constructive anger*). This differs from the above free expression method in that we express ourselves in a controlled and dignified manner and hope that others are willing to listen to our point of view.

Therefore, we can appreciate that holding in our anger, and not expressing it, is not a worthwhile idea. Free expression of anger also creates a whole complex of other counterproductive problems. Further, we have noted that creative aggression seems a more workable solution but that it still shares some of the same problems. According to Ellis (1977), another alternative, that of "*Christian forgiveness,*" involves the "turning of the other cheek." But in this aggressive, often hostile world in which we live, this seems somewhat impractical.

According to Ellis (1977), anger begets anger. Therefore, the most practical solution in dealing with our anger within is that we need to become *annoyed and irritated,* so that we can become more effective at solving problems. We get angry, then we try to fix the problem. Then we get upset with our own anger, and now we develop a problem with the anger and its consequences. When we become angry, we either "let it out" or "hold it in." A third choice is to become *annoyed and irritated;* thus we can solve problems. Ellis and

Harper (1975) suggest that many people create irrational beliefs about what we should and should not do regarding anger. Research shows that when some people become angry, they need to reach closure immediately. For others, it is necessary to be alone, take time out, and work out the anger for themselves. Actually, in our culture we do not seem to have the best vocabulary to define those intense feelings we identify as anger. When people become angry, they often say, "You did that," rather than, "I get annoyed" when you do that. Anger comes from a belief that the world should not be the way it is and should be the way I want it to be. This is really an acknowledgment of the fact that all people have the freedom of will to choose to behave badly. If people do not have free will, then moral philosophy need not exist. When people behave badly, they have that right. No matter how many laws exist, one can never take away a person's free will. Ellis's school of thought suggests that we acknowledge and accept what others are by seeing these differences and becoming annoyed and irritated with these differences (Dryden & DiGiuseppe, 1990; Walen, DiGiuseppe, & Wessler, 1980). This *annoyance and irritation* on our part is often helpful in managing anger, for it helps us attain a balance (see Box 5.1).

Box 5.1 Tips on Managing Anger Based on Eastern Philosophy

Following are some helpful behavioral tips for managing anger within oneself. These are based on Eastern thoughts. We may want to reflect on some of these, and if we find any of these tips helpful we must adopt these in our lives.

- *Introspection:* In any situation that makes us angry, there is always a component of our own responsibility. Therefore, we must always reflect on our contribution in triggering the anger. Any time we get angry, we should always try to find our mistake, no matter how little or trivial our contribution might have been. When we are angry or immediately after we have given way to anger it is often not a good time for such "soul searching." However, once the mind has become a little calmer and at the same time not much time has elapsed since we got angry (not so much that we have forgotten all about it) is often a good time for performing this introspection. We should be critical of our own behavior and give the "benefit of the doubt" to the other party. Also we should analyze the situation from the other person's point of view—we should try to step into the other person's shoes and look at the event triggering our anger from his or her perspective. Keeping these points in mind will help us decipher our own contribution toward anger.

Box 5.1 Tips on Managing Anger Based on Eastern Philosophy (cont'd)

- *Apologizing and Determining to Rectify Our Contribution:* Once we have identified our contribution in the situation that made us angry, if possible we should make it a point to apologize to the other person for our contribution without getting into any further argument. After apologizing, or if apologizing is not possible, we should make a conscious effort *not to repeat the same mistake* when we encounter a similar cue for action. We must repeat in our mind that we must not give way to anger next time when we are confronted with a similar situation. *Often in life, we keep on repeating the same mistakes again and again.* Reflection on the root cause in any situation that triggers our anger oftentimes helps us decipher these repetitive patterns of mistakes. Developing a conscious awareness about these repetitive mistakes and fortifying the mind in dealing with them is often a helpful way to reduce the anger within ourselves in future encounters with similar triggers.

- *Understanding That Not Everything Can Be Changed, Fixed, or Altered:* Often our anger is directed toward another person or situation that cannot be changed, fixed, or altered. Understanding this very important reality of life and channeling our energies toward changing our own modifiable behaviors (which are frequently the only components that can be changed) is often a helpful strategy at making us less angry.

- *Letting Go:* In present-day society, we have become overtly competitive in our disposition. We want to win at all cost, compete with others, covet the same things that others have, and imagine that possessions will make us happier. Often these kinds of expectations are at the root of our anger. Remembering that life is not about competing with anyone but pursuing a journey of self-realization is indeed helpful in reducing anger in our lives.

* * * * *

Thoughts for Reflection 5.1
What Anger Is

• An emotional response	Anger is an emotional reaction that normally happens in response to an unfulfilled desire, an unmet expectation, and an unimagined consequence.
• A warning signal	Anger helps us to identify that something is wrong and is preventing us from achieving our goals.
• A way to new learning	Usually anger facilitates our power of reflection and opens a door to new learning, provided that we have an open mind and are willing to learn.
• A normal feeling	Anger is a normal response that all of us experience, and it is not abnormal to be angry.
• Healthy within limits	Since anger is a feeling, if it is contained and not let out as a behavior, then it serves to release pent-up emotions. However, we need not deny, repress, or suppress anger for it to be healthy.
• A protective mechanism	Anger helps all living beings to protect themselves from unconducive surroundings and situations.
• Useful within limits	Anger helps us in setting interactive boundaries with people around us. It serves an important purpose in letting others appreciate what we like and what we dislike.

* * * * *

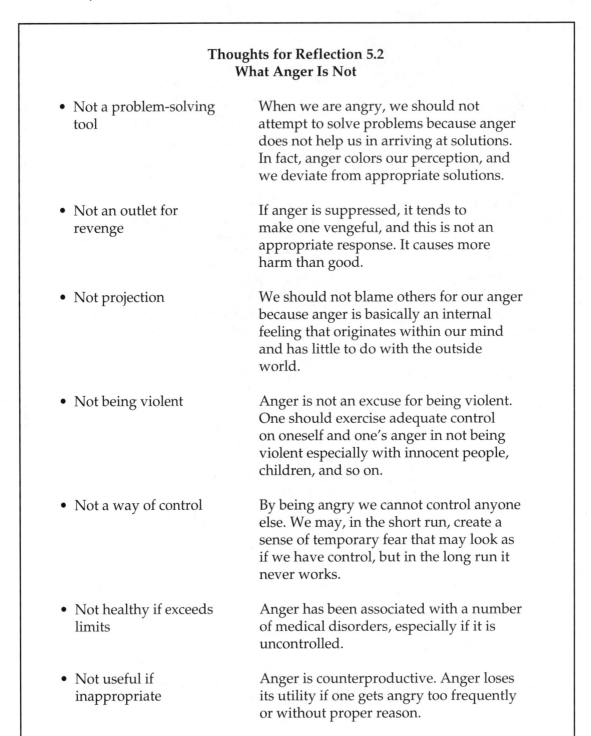

Thoughts for Reflection 5.2
What Anger Is Not

• Not a problem-solving tool	When we are angry, we should not attempt to solve problems because anger does not help us in arriving at solutions. In fact, anger colors our perception, and we deviate from appropriate solutions.
• Not an outlet for revenge	If anger is suppressed, it tends to make one vengeful, and this is not an appropriate response. It causes more harm than good.
• Not projection	We should not blame others for our anger because anger is basically an internal feeling that originates within our mind and has little to do with the outside world.
• Not being violent	Anger is not an excuse for being violent. One should exercise adequate control on oneself and one's anger in not being violent especially with innocent people, children, and so on.
• Not a way of control	By being angry we cannot control anyone else. We may, in the short run, create a sense of temporary fear that may look as if we have control, but in the long run it never works.
• Not healthy if exceeds limits	Anger has been associated with a number of medical disorders, especially if it is uncontrolled.
• Not useful if inappropriate	Anger is counterproductive. Anger loses its utility if one gets angry too frequently or without proper reason.

* * * * *

Anger and Stress: The Connection

As we have shown in Chapter 1, the stress response has two components: *fight* and *flight*. The fight component of the stress response is a naturally occurring event, which is also responsible for angry behavior. Signs of anger and stress are interchangeable. Both anger and stress lead to anxiety, sleeplessness, uncontrolled thinking, brooding, restlessness, irritability, and so on. Along with these manifestations come headaches, muscle tension, peptic ulcers, and other stress-related problems. More dangerous are the reactions that we cannot feel (Eliot & Breo, 1989).

Another important dimension in the context of anger and stress is our personality. In people with Type A personalities, it appears that hostility and anger may be the key (Friedman & Rosenman, 1959, 1974). We have already seen in Chapter 1 that people with Type A personalities experience greater stress and the negative sequelae associated with stress. Coronary heart disease and essential hypertension are two important diseases in particular that have been linked with anger. Some psychologists believe that hypertensives keep their blood pressure elevated by constantly suppressing their anger. According to Tavris (1982), "Release the anger and blood pressure should fall."

Anger also involves the feeling of pain and/or injury to oneself. If we personalize anger, we become fearful and anxious, feel cornered, become further angered, and lose control. This "loss of control" causes us to form judgments and make assumptions, and further escalates our feeling of anger. In order to maintain balance and prevent anger from escalating, we need to preserve our self-worth, keep things in perspective, not unduly feed our fears, and *decide* to be in control of ourselves. Thus we reserve judgment and are able to maintain a problem-solving attitude. Anger is useful as a *signal* in which a "warning light" causes us to take action. As a solution, anger rarely helps, for it adds fuel to the fire, heats up the problem, and may cause inappropriate action.

Expectations control our reactions to anger. That which we usually expect and which does not happen acts as a "triggering event" and causes a reaction to which we seek a solution. The first time an expectation is not met, we have no idea how to approach this situation, so we think about what to do. If our solution seems to work, we try it out again in future situations. Once we are sure our solution works, we no longer wonder about whether it will work, and so we stop thinking about it and just do it. In this way, a habit is formed. If we have learned to respond by getting angry, then we will respond in that way irrespective of what the consequences will be. As time passes, reflection on the consequences decreases further and further. We also remind ourselves less and less about what it is that we are to do. This is an efficient way to operate provided that our solution is really a good solution. In the case of anger, it is not a good solution. What really happens is that it causes a "fire," and we have to face the harmful consequences. This response needs to be changed. The following steps are to be considered in effecting this change:

1. Recognize and admit that our old solution is not working.

2. Use the old reaction as a cue to start a new search for a new solution.

3. Activate our thinking to identify the expectations upon which we are basing our reactions, and begin to examine them critically.

4. Examine the validity of our expectations, reject those we find are not true or helpful, and replace them with ones that are.

5. With new expectations the response will change.

6. Keep reinforcing these new expectations over and over again.

In order to manage the anger within, we need to identify situations in which we are likely to be angry. Then we have to look for the *cues* for anger that trigger an event. Unfulfilled and unrealistic expectations are often at the root of most anger. An understanding of these is helpful in reducing anger. Next we have to analyze the *costs* and *benefits* that come after our anger has subsided and the event is over. Managing anger basically involves modifying these cues and consequences, and finding effective replacements for the anger.

Therefore, the first step in managing anger is to find out where you are with anger in your personal life. Worksheet 5.1 has been designed to help you enhance this understanding, and Worksheet 5.2 helps you manage anger.

Thoughts for Reflection 5.3
Points to Ponder

- The troubles of our proud and angry dust
  Are from eternity, and shall not fail.
  Bear them we can, and if we can we must.
  Shoulder the sky, my lad, and drink your ale.

  —A. E. HOUSMAN

- Anger is never without an argument, but seldom with a good.

  —GEORGE SAVILE, MARQUIS OF HALIFAX

- Anger is one of the sinews of the soul. Anger makes a rich man hated and a poor man scorned.

  —THOMAS FULLER

- Where it concerns himself, Who's angry at a slander makes it true.

  —BEN JONSON

- He that is slow to anger is better than the mighty; and he that ruleth his spirit than he that taketh a city.

  —PROVERBS 16:32

- Anger makes dull men witty, but it keeps them poor.

  —QUEEN ELIZABETH I

- Anger is a weed; hate is the tree.

  —ST. AUGUSTINE

- In the depth of winter I finally learned that within me lay an invincible summer.

  —ALBERT CAMUS

- Anyone can become angry—that is easy. But to be angry with the right person, to the right degree, at the right time, for the right purpose, and in the right way—that is not easy.

  —ARISTOTLE

* * * * *

Worksheet 5.1
Self-Assessment of Anger

Respond to the following questions honestly. Responses will serve as a means of feedback for your own improvement in managing anger.

1. Is anger a problem for me? ____ Yes ____ No ____ Not sure

2. How do I know when I am angry?

____

____

____

____

____

____

3. How do I feel inside when I am angry?

____

____

____

____

____

____

4. What do I do about my anger?

____

____

____

____

____

____

Worksheet 5.1 Self-Assessment of Anger (cont'd)

5. Describe the last time when you got angry. At what or with whom were you angry? How did this affect you?

____

____

____

____

____

6. Analyze your reasons for becoming angry.

____

____

____

____

____

7. Indicate any problems created by your anger.

____

____

____

____

____

8. List other ways you could have solved the problem without getting angry.

____

____

____

____

____

FEEDBACK ON WORKSHEET 5.1

Worksheet 5.1 helps you to acquire a greater insight into the situations and persons with whom you become angry. If you can identify the situations that cause your anger and the various negative consequences that you have to face as a result of your anger, you can become more motivated to change your behavior. This enhanced awareness is the basis of and the first step toward changing your response to anger.

* * * * *

Worksheet 5.2
Managing Your Anger

This worksheet is designed to help you deal with your anger in a more productive way. Seek out a quiet place to reflect upon and respond to the following statements.

1. Identify a situation in which you have expressed anger inappropriately. Analyze your goals and/or desired expectations. Then break the situation down into steps. Examine at which step the anger became apparent.

   Situation:

   ____

   ____

   ____

   ____

   Goals/desired expectations:

   ____

   ____

   Steps in the event:

   ____

   ____

   ____

   ____

   ____

2. Describe the benefits that this anger had.

   ____

   ____

   ____

Worksheet 5.2 Managing Your Anger (cont'd)

3. Did the anger cost you anything or cause any harm?

____

____

____

____

4. Do the costs outweigh the benefits? ____ Yes ____ No

5. What alternative step(s) could you have taken instead of the one in which you got angry and still met your goal/desired expectation?

____

____

____

6. What were the barriers that prevented you from adopting this alternative step?

____

____

____

____

____

7. How can you overcome these barriers in the future?

____

____

____

____

____

* * * * *

Dealing with an Angry Person

I. Transactional Analysis

Eric Berne (1967) described a technique called Transactional Analysis (TA), a method for understanding interpersonal transactions. Transactions are defined as units of social intercourse.

An understanding of the basics of this method will enhance our skills to deal with anger within ourself, as well as relate better with an angry person. According to Transactional Analysis, the various aspects of our personalities can be classified into three states:

a. *The Child Ego State.* The child ego state is the state in which we enter the world. Within the child state are three dimensions: (1) the *free child,* which is inquisitive, wants to have fun, be liked, and be admired; (2) the *rebellious child,* which has been acquired because of certain experiences in our childhood and rebels against domination; and (3) the *manipulative child,* which has developed as a result of our learning some manipulative behavior in order to get our needs fulfilled as children. An angry person is almost always in the child ego state—rebellious or manipulative, and this ego state needs to be addressed first.

b. *The Parent Ego State.* The parent ego state is the repository for events as we perceived them in the early years of our lives, up to five years of age. These recordings or parent tapes owe their origin to our parents and other significant people during our childhood who told us what to do and what not to do. These messages are resolved without editing and include all prohibitions, admonitions, and rules set by example or stated. The parent ego state has two parts: (1) the *critical parent,* which results in pronouncement of most imperatives like "you should," "you must," and "you ought to," and (2) the *nurturing or caring parent,* which sympathizes, listens, encourages, and exhibits care and love.

c. *The Adult Ego State.* The adult ego state is not synonymous with maturity. However, this is the rational part of us and operates on data gathering and analysis. It is unemotional and helps us look at things through facts and objectivity.

The most interesting aspect of this theory is that all of us possess these stages within ourselves. What happens with anger is that we transcend into the child ego state. However, sometimes we may not appear childlike because we have camouflaged our feelings as either "critical parents," "caring parents," or "rational adults." If masquerading as a "critical parent," we tend to use what we *should* have done or *ought* to be doing. In the mask of "caring parent" we tend to be sarcastic. In the mask of a "rational adult" ego state, we may try to give justification and rationalization that may actually be biased, and underneath might be a burning inferno. Besides other emotions like worry and fear, bereavement may also appear like anger, but needs to be addressed in a different way.

With this understanding it is clear that in anger a person is in a "child" ego state and this fact should be addressed first. It can be tackled by a *"caring parent" response followed by a "rational adult" response.* The problem occurs when we respond as a "critical parent" or evoke our "child" ego state or move directly to the adult stage bypassing the "caring parent." These responses do not extinguish anger but only make it flare up further. Evoking a "caring parent" response helps angry people to be at ease and feel that their behavior has been addressed. When this is followed by a "rational adult" response, then understanding by an angry person of his or her "mistake(s)" is achieved. In this way this approach helps to disarm any angry person.

For example, a fellow student or fellow worker becomes angry with us on some event and stops speaking. If we do not speak to that person it is likely to add to the existing anger. However, if we approach that person with a caring attitude and inquiries about the reason for his or her anger, it is likely that he or she will narrate the event from his or her perspective. Having reestablished this rapport and understood the problem from the other person's perspective we can *rationally* analyze the situation and thus resolve the anger between both of us.

II. The "Time-out" Procedure

Often, when we are angry, we do not think. In order to reactivate our thinking, we need to put aside everything in which we are engaged and find time to reflect and introspect. The "Time-out" Procedure detailed in this section (Coursol & Veenstra, 1986) provides us with this opportunity to reflect upon our actions, then accordingly change them. It consists of the following steps:

a. *Stop:* We have to immediately put a stop to our conventional behavior. This implies that we can no longer respond by getting angry at situations in which we got angry earlier. This determination to "stop" is the first step in the "Time-out" Procedure.

b. *Think:* Having stopped our conventional response, we need to think about a new approach in dealing with situations that may potentiate anger. Think about this new way by identifying and describing the new skills that will be required. Also think about the approaches and possible barriers in acquiring these new skills.

c. *Act:* Overcome the cognitive barriers (i.e., faulty beliefs and expectations) that stand in our way to implement the new way. Having overcome the barriers, act on the new way by practicing the new skills.

The effectiveness of the "Time-out" Procedure is based upon the other person's view of the position we have taken. A person's perception is a factor here in that once we attempt to practice the "Time-out" Procedure, it is up to the other person to react to us. An angry person wants to get his or her point across to us. This provides that person with a relief from their sense of injustice. This also gives hope that the problem-solving process has started. What an angry person usually gets is a counterattack explaining why he or she was wrong. Since the "defense of self" is a priority, an angry person does not listen (Coursol & Veenstra, 1986). What an angry person does in response is defend the self and attack more intensely. His or her anger is increased because of the pain felt of not getting through. The angry person becomes apprehensive that the problem will continue unsolved. In the "Time-out" Procedure (Coursol & Veenstra, 1986) options that are helpful when listening to an angry person consist of the following:

- *Reflective or Empathic Listening.* "What you are saying is . . ." In this approach we are serving as a mirror, acknowledging what the other person is saying but not putting out our own view as a target. Our own viewpoint is preserved and set aside from consideration.
- *Possible Agreement or Fogging.* "Let me think about that . . ." In this approach we acknowledge that the other person might be on target, but we are not committing ourselves definitely. It is important to follow through on problem solving so the other person will not see it as a stall.
- *Actual Agreement or Admitting That We Are Wrong.* "You are right, it was wrong for me to . . ." In this approach we acknowledge that the other person is on target and admit that we are wrong and at fault. If we don't really believe we are wrong, this will only "stuff" and not solve the problem.
- *Negative Inquiry or Inviting Further Criticism.* "Are there other things I do that hurt you?" In this approach we give an opportunity to have the other person aim at the target. This must be done genuinely.

This valuable technique, which has been shown to manage anger effectively, is the "Time-out" Procedure as shown in Figure 5.1.

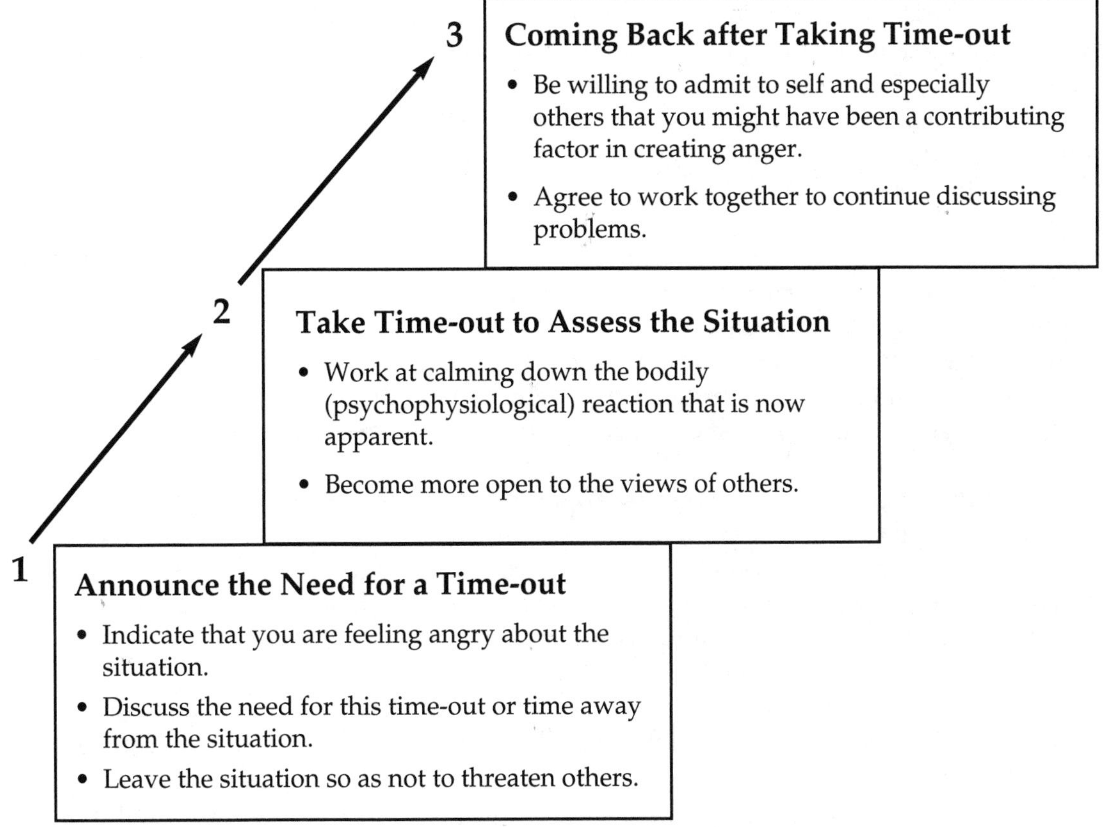

3
Coming Back after Taking Time-out
• Be willing to admit to self and especially others that you might have been a contributing factor in creating anger.
• Agree to work together to continue discussing problems.
2
Take Time-out to Assess the Situation
• Work at calming down the bodily (psychophysiological) reaction that is now apparent.
• Become more open to the views of others.
1
Announce the Need for a Time-out
• Indicate that you are feeling angry about the situation.
• Discuss the need for this time-out or time away from the situation.
• Leave the situation so as not to threaten others.

Figure 5.1 The "Time-out" Procedure

III. The "Upset" Philosophy

According to Myers and Nance (1991) angry people are usually "upset." Moreover, we also become "upset" when we have to deal with an angry person. We can cope with an angry person if we can identify and understand the specific incident that triggered the anger. We will also have success in preventing another person from becoming angry if we understand the kinds of situations that are likely to be anger provoking.

Anger is the result of many factors, including the triggering or precipitating situation, our past experiences, individual responses to experiences, and idiosyncrasies. Understanding what creates anger in another person is often helpful both in planning preventive strategies and in deciding how to handle anger once it occurs. Therefore, we have to examine the situation of the other person. We have to step into the shoes of the other person and then look at the situation from his or her angle.

Myers and Nance (1991) have identified several triggering factors and events, as follows:

1. *Dependency.* Usually a feeling of dependence on another person, object, or thing can lead to increased anger. Anger is especially accentuated when we are intimately dependent and cannot find alternatives to our dependency. A person with such feelings can be helped by providing enough *choices* and helping that person to *become more independent.*

2. *Authority.* Authority normally comes by position, expertise, or wealth. Oftentimes authority makes a person inappropriately authoritarian. People who are authoritarian tend to utilize their authority in a manner that provokes anger. It is the way they say things that creates anger in others. It may not be *what* they say but *how* they say it that precipitates anger. Therefore, one needs to be very careful in how one is presenting a point of view and using one's authority.

3. *Unclear Limits.* Some of us want and seek direction in how we perform our tasks. These directions can come from our parents, our peers, our teachers, our employers, our colleagues, our spouses, and so on. When these directions are unclear, confusing, or dualistic, then they lead to anger and frustration. Anger originating from this type of unclarity can be dealt with by setting specific directions and limits. If these directions come from within ourselves, then greater autonomy and control can be achieved in dealing with anger.

4. *Complexity.* Many situations are apparently complicated, intricate, and complex. If we get stuck in the complexity, then we are prone to get angry. This type of anger can be tackled, simplifying the process by breaking it down into smaller parts or steps. Breaking down any complicated event into smaller parts or steps often simplifies the process. We need to constantly remember that life is essentially a simple process.

5. *Prior Unresolved Conflict.* Past events are an important source of our anger, especially events on which we have not reached closure or which have not been resolved amicably. These events and associated anger keep surfacing again and again. Until and unless these conflicts are completely resolved, sublimation of anger cannot result. We need to put our mind and effort toward resolving conflicts that we can resolve. We need to strengthen our mind to "forgive" and "forget" the conflicts over which we have no control.

6. *Communication Problems.* We have seen in Chapter 4 that poor, ineffective, and marginal communication often leads to stress and anger. If we are not able to communicate effectively, this failure causes anger and frustration in us as well as others. This poor communication can result from a number of causes. Some of these causes may pertain to us, while others may pertain to others. Though we cannot do much about how others communicate, we can certainly improve upon our own communication, especially when this miscommunication is an intended one, for inexplicable reasons, on our part. As far as possible we should try to identify these reasons, overcome them, and make our communication as clear and effective as possible.

7. *Conflict of Interest.* People have different ideas and interests. Sometimes when a task needs to be achieved, these differences tend to be mutually conflicting. This conflict can be a source of anger and frustration. Therefore, all potential conflicts need to be resolved. Thoughts for Reflection 5.4 and 5.5 provide some suggestions for resolving conflicts.

Thoughts for Reflection 5.4
Five Conflict-Handling Orientations

Conflict-Handling Orientation	*Appropriate Situations*
1. Competition	• When quick, decisive action is vital • On the important issues where unpopular actions need implementing • On issues vital to the organization's welfare and when you know you're right • Against people who take advantage of noncompetitive behavior
2. Collaboration	• To find an integrative solution when both sets of concerns are too important to be compromised • When your objective is to learn • To merge insights from people with different perspectives

Thoughts for Reflection 5.4 Five Conflict-Handling Orientations (cont'd)

Conflict-Handling Orientation	*Appropriate Situations*
	• To gain commitment by incorporating concerns into a consensus • To work through feelings that have interfered with a relationship
3. Avoidance	• When an issue is trivial, or more important issues are pressing • When you perceive no chance of satisfying your concerns • When potential disruption outweighs the benefits of resolution • To let people cool down and regain perspective • When gathering information supersedes immediate decision • When others can resolve the conflict more effectively • When issues seem tangential or symptomatic of other issues
4. Accommodate	• When you find you are wrong to allow better position to be heard, to learn, and to show your reasonableness • When issues are more important to others than yourself to satisfy others and maintain cooperation • To build social credits for later issues • To minimize loss when you are outmatched and losing • When harmony and stability are especially important • To allow subordinates to develop by learning from mistakes
5. Compromise	• When goals are important but not worth the effort or potential disruption of more assertive modes • When opponents with equal power are committed to mutually exclusive goals • To achieve temporary settlements to complex issues • To arrive at expedient solutions under time pressure • As a backup when collaboration or competition is unsuccessful

Note: From "Toward multidimensional values in teaching: The example of conflict behaviors" by K. W. Thomas, July 1977, *Academy of Management Review*, p. 487. Copyright 1977 by Academy of Management Review. Reprinted by permission.

* * * * *

Thoughts for Reflection 5.5
Resolving Conflicts by Managing Anger

Once you have some idea of what anger is and what causes it, you are ready to think about a process for defusing anger in other people. Some methods for dealing with anger include these:

- *Listening.* We really have to work at listening. Listen for the content, the feelings, and those things with which you can agree. Listen without your critical parent, without personalizing, and without counterattacking. Cover your hot buttons, and cover your rear.
- *Acknowledge Feelings.* Acknowledge that the other person is angry. Do not try to talk him or her out of feeling angry. Simply understand what the person is experiencing.
- *Agreeing.* State areas of agreement. This method involves a different mindset. It means that we are not listening to catch the other person when they exaggerate, get confused, or overreact. Rather, we are listening for those things with which we can agree.
- *Getting Agreement on the Problem.* It is important to get some agreement on the problem.
- *Finding Solutions.* Agreeing first on the problem, identifying possible solutions, and then agreeing on one solution.
- *Closing.* "Is there anything else I can do?" "Are you feeling satisfied at the outcome?" "Let me know what else I can do." Thank the person for letting you know that they were angry. It helps to keep things straight between you. When you know what the problem is, a better chance of solving it exists.

Note: From *The upset book,* 2nd ed. (p. 103–131), by P. Myers and D. Nance, 1991. Wichita, KS: Mac Press. Copyright 1991 by Pennie Myers and Don Nance. Adapted by permission.

* * * * *

IV. Active Listening

An important factor in managing anger is the ability to listen actively. Active listening is an intervention that addresses our interaction with others (Steinmetz, Blankenship, Brown, Hall, & Miller, 1980). This is an effective yet simple tool for managing anger and thereby reducing stress. Its applicability has multifarious uses.

First, active listening is a *diagnostic tool.* It helps one to identify and pinpoint the cause or reason for the other person's anger. Second, active listening is a *disarming device* that helps the angry person to appropriately "let out" his or her feelings. Third, active listening provides an opportunity to seek *clarification,* which is an important component for resolving anger. Fourth, active listening aids to *rationalize,* develop *clear thinking,* and *communicate effectively* in order to mutually resolve anger. Finally, active listening helps the angry person to preserve his or her *dignity* and not express anger in an undignified manner.

Worksheet 5.3 has been designed to help you deal more effectively with an angry person through active listening. Since this worksheet involves role-playing, it cannot be completed alone and requires the cooperation of a partner.

Worksheet 5.3
Learning Active Listening

In order to practice active listening, you will require the cooperation of a partner. This activity involves role-playing and sharpening your skills to listen actively. Ask your partner to imagine a situation in which he or she was or will be angry with you. Let him or her imagine that situation mentally. You, as well as your partner, will have to work at this role-play. Following are some of the guidelines for you to work on.

Self	**Partner**
• *Direct questioning:* Start probing the reasons for the partner's anger in a calm and controlled manner.	• Since you are angry, you may choose to respond or not respond.
• *Rationalizing:* Try to understand the partner's feelings. Also try to understand the reasons and explanations for this behavior in your own mind.	• Act out the way you actually feel.
• *Clarifying:* You may want to seek clarification on your partner's feelings and responses.	• Behave the way you feel.
• *Supporting:* As far as possible try to support your partner's viewpoint. This may be difficult, but you should attempt to do it.	• You may choose whether or not to yield to the responses.

FEEDBACK ON WORKSHEET 5.3

Both you and your partner need to focus on the way you are feeling now. Has the anger been resolved? If so, discuss the reasons. If not, discuss why not. You may want to write out in the space below some of your learnings from this experience.

You may want to reinforce these learnings from time to time so that they become a part of your behavior, and then you can deal with an angry person more effectively. Your partner may want to change roles with you and improve his or her ability to deal with angry people.

* * * * *

Thoughts for Reflection 5.6
Calming Reminders

1. Do not take anger personally. Maintain a sense of self-worth. Ask yourself:
   - "Are they having a rough day?"
   - "Is this really directed to me?"
   - "Are they just criticizing my behavior, not my being?"

2. Keep anger in perspective. Do not feed your fears. Tell yourself:
   - "Relax, you can make it through this."
   - "It is not going to be the end of the world."
   - "It is not that bad."

3. Decide to be in control of yourself. Repeat to yourself:
   - "I shall not let the anger control me."
   - "I can and will control the anger."

4. Do not be judgmental. Ask yourself:
   - "Do I need to attribute reasons?"
   - "Am I expecting too much in this situation?"
   - "Can anyone always win?"

5. Maintain a problem-solving attitude. Ask yourself:
   - "Do I have an open mind?"
   - "What are the alternatives?"

* * * * *

Thoughts for Reflection 5.7
The Value of "I" Messages

If you start a statement with an "I," it implies you are owning responsibility. If you start a statement with "you," that implies that you are shifting responsibility to the other person. Every "you" message can be turned into an "I" message. Then it becomes a nonblaming statement about one's own self. Of course, you cannot always talk in calm "I" messages all the time. There is no distinct advantage in using "I" messages for all situations. If your goal is to let the other person know that you are angry, you can do it in your own personal style, and your style may do the job. If, however, your goal is to break a pattern in an important relationship and/or to develop a stronger sense of self that you can bring to all your relationships, it is essential that you learn to translate your anger into clear, nonblaming statements about yourself, that is, "I" statements (Lerner, 1985).

* * * * *

Stress Management Principle 5

Balancing your anger balances your life.

Summary Points

- Unmanaged anger is harmful to self and others.
- Anger is an internal *feeling* that, if not managed, results in aggression, which is a destructive *behavior.*
- Denying, repressing, or even freely expressing anger is often harmful.
- In order to manage anger within ourselves, through Rational Emotive Therapy as described by Albert Ellis, we need to become *annoyed* and *irritated.* This annoyance and irritation help us to attain balance with anger.
- Unfulfilled and unrealistic expectations are at the root of anger. An understanding of these often leads to decreased anger.
- Transactional Analysis, first described by Eric Berne, is a useful technique in dealing with an angry person.
- According to Transactional Analysis, our personalities have three ego states: "child" (free, rebellious, manipulative), "parent" (critical, caring), and "adult" (rational).
- A "caring parent" response followed by a "rational adult," is often helpful in extinguishing the anger of an angry person.
- The "Time-out" Procedure, or giving oneself adequate time to reflect and introspect on dealing with an angry person, is often a helpful approach.
- The "Upset" philosophy, described by Myers and Nance, recognizes several triggering factors for anger: dependency, authority, unclear limits, complexity, prior unresolved conflict, communication problems, and conflict of interest.
- Five conflict-handling orientations are competition, collaboration, avoidance, accommodation, and compromise.
- Active listening is an effective tool to disarm any angry person. It involves direct questioning, rationalizing, clarifying, and supporting.

References and Further Readings

Berne, E. (1967). *Transactional analysis.* New York: Harper College.

Coursol, D., & Veenstra, G. (1986). *Anger control.* Unpublished manuscript, University of Kansas School of Medicine, Wichita.

Davis, M., Eshelman, E. R., & McKay, M. (1982). *The relaxation and stress reduction workbook* (2nd ed.). Oakland, CA: New Harbinger.

Dryden, W., & DiGiuseppe, R. (1990). *A primer on rational-emotive therapy.* Champaign, IL: Research Press.

Eliot, R. S., & Breo, D. L. (1989). *Is it worth dying for? How to make stress work for you—not against you.* New York: Bantam.

Ellis, A. (1975). *How to live with a neurotic.* North Hollywood, CA: Wilshire.

Ellis, A. (1977). *Anger: How to live with and without it.* Secaucus, NJ: Citadel Press.

Ellis, A., & Harper, R. A. (1975). *A new guide to rational living.* North Hollywood, CA: Wilshire.

Friedman, M., & Rosenman, R. H. (1959). Association of specific overt behavior pattern with blood and cardiovascular findings: Blood clotting time, incidence of arcus senilis, and clinical coronary artery disease. *Journal of the American Medical Association, 169,* 1286–1296.

Friedman, M., & Rosenman, R. H. (1974). *Type A behavior and your heart.* New York: Fawcett Crest.

Greenberg, J. S. (1999). *Comprehensive stress management* (6th. ed.). Boston: William C. Brown/McGraw-Hill.

Lerner, H. G. (1985). *The dance of anger.* New York: Harper & Row.

Myers, P., & Nance, D. (1991). *The upset book* (2nd ed.). Wichita, KS: Mac Press.

Smith, J. C. (1993). *Creative stress management: The 1-2-3 cope system.* Englewood Cliffs, NJ: Prentice-Hall.

Steinmetz, J., Blankenship, J., Brown, L., Hall, D., & Miller, G. (1980). *Managing stress before it manages you.* Palo Alto, CA: Bull.

Tavris, C. (1982). *Anger: The misunderstood emotion.* New York: Simon & Schuster.

Thomas, K. W. (1977). Toward multidimensional values in teaching: The example of conflict behaviors. *Academy of Management Review,* 487.

Walen, S. R., DiGiuseppe, R., & Wessler, R. L. (1980). *A practitioner's guide to rational-emotive therapy.* New York: Oxford University Press.

CHAPTER 6

Coping with Anxiety

To John Dryden of Chesterton

How blessed is he, who leads a country life,
Unvex'd with anxious cares, and void of strife!
Who studying peace, and shunning civil rage,
Enjoy'd his youth, and now enjoys his age:
All who deserve his love, he makes his own;
And, to be lov'd himself, needs only to be known.

—*John Dryden*

What Is Anxiety?

Anxiety is an inevitable part of life. Inherent in anxiety are two components—inefficiency and fear. *Inefficiency* is the loss of one's mental alertness and inability to gear the mind toward problem solving. To *fear* is to imagine that one's own actions always have bad or painful consequences, or to imagine only possible adverse events (Maharishi, 1989). Greenberg (1999) has described anxiety, operationally, as an unrealistic fear resulting in physiological arousal and accompanied by the behavioral signs of escape or avoidance. When this feeling of anxiety becomes uncontrolled or excessive, then it knocks one down. Various mental disorders are associated with excessive anxiety. Generalized Anxiety Disorder is characterized by unrealistic or excessive anxiety and worry about life situations. Some of the symptoms of this disorder are as follows (*Diagnostic and Statistical Manual of Mental Disorders*—DSM IV, 1994):

1. Trembling, twitching, feeling shaky
2. Muscle tension, aches, soreness
3. Restlessness
4. Easy fatiguability
5. Shortness of breath
6. Palpitations, feeling of heart beating faster
7. Sweating
8. Dryness of mouth

9. Dizziness, light-headedness
10. Nausea
11. Flushes
12. Frequent urination
13. Trouble in swallowing, "lump in throat"
14. Feeling "keyed up" or "on edge"
15. Difficulty concentrating
16. Irritability
17. Trouble falling or staying asleep

In some rural areas and subpopulations of the United States, patients use unique expressions to describe anxiety like "I got the churnings," "I'm uptight," or "I am always freaking out" (Shader & Greenblatt, 1993).

Another type of anxiety disorder is panic disorder. The key symptoms associated with panic attacks are these (DSM IV, 1994):

1. Shortness of breath, smothering sensation
2. Dizziness, unsteady feelings, or faintness
3. Palpitations
4. Trembling, shaking
5. Sweating
6. Choking
7. Nausea, abdominal distress
8. Depersonalization, derealization
9. Numbness, tingling sensations
10. Flushes
11. Chest pain
12. Fear of dying
13. Fear of going crazy or doing something uncontrolled

Panic disorders may occur alone or in conjunction with a secondary syndrome termed "agoraphobia," which is defined as a fear of being in places or situations from which escape might be difficult or embarrassing or in which help might not be available in the event of a panic attack. Affected persons usually restrict their travel or need a companion when they are away from home or other familiar places. The severity of avoidance behavior can range from mild, where there is distress, to severe, where the person is completely homebound.

Some other anxiety disorders include the following (DSM IV, 1994):

1. *Specific phobias,* which consist of excessive or unreasonable fear of a specific object or situation (for example, elevators, flying, heights, or some type of animal).
2. *Social phobias,* which include a marked and persistent fear of social or performance situations (for example, public speaking, entering a room full of strangers, or using a public restroom).
3. *Obsessive compulsive disorders* (OCD), which consist of obsessions and compulsions. Obsessions are recurrent and persistent thoughts, impulses, or images that are intrusive and inappropriate and cause anxiety. Compulsions are urgent repetitive behaviors such as hand washing, counting, or repeatedly checking to make sure that some dreaded event will not occur (for example, checking that all doors are locked and then checking again and again).
4. *Post-traumatic stress disorder* (PTSD) in which a person has been exposed to an event that involved actual or threatened death or serious injury, and the person reacted with intense fear, helplessness, or horror. In the disorder the person persistently reexperiences the event through recollections or dreams or a sudden feeling as if it were recurring.

Besides anxiety sometimes a person may also manifest depression. The classical signs and symptoms of depression include presence of five or more of the following (DSM IV, 1994):

1. Depressed mood most of the day, nearly every day
2. Diminished interest or pleasure in most activities
3. Significant changes in body weight or appetite (increased or decreased)
4. Insomnia or hypersomnia nearly every day
5. Psychomotor agitation (increased activity) or retardation (decreased activity)
6. Fatigue or loss of energy
7. Feelings of worthlessness or excessive guilt
8. Diminished ability to think or concentrate
9. Recurrent thoughts of death or suicide attempt or plan to commit suicide

Population-based surveys about emotional disorders in the United States have revealed a one-year period prevalence of anxiety among adults between 5 and 15 percent and panic disorders between 1 and 2 percent (Regier et al., 1988).

These are, however, representations of pathological conditions that require treatment with benzodiazepines and other drugs. In this chapter we will learn about mechanisms that can prevent these conditions from occurring. Prevention requires systematic and regular practice in order to cope with worrying and anxiety so that these feelings do not get out of proportion and result in disorders. By learning these practical techniques, one can reduce worrying and anxiety and maintain long-lasting health and happiness in life.

Before you proceed to learn these techniques, take the Taylor Manifest Anxiety Scale in Worksheet 6.1, which measures the degree to which you manifest anxiety.

Thoughts for Reflection 6.1
When You Worry, Think!

- Why do you worry unnecessarily? Who is it that you fear? Who can kill you? The soul is immortal.

- Whatever has happened has been good. Whatever is happening is good. Whatever will happen will be good. Do not regret the past. Do not worry about the future.

- What is it that you have lost? What did you bring that you have lost? What did you create that is now no more? You did not bring anything to this world. Whatever you took you took here. You came empty-handed and you will go empty-handed. Whatever belongs to you today belonged to someone else yesterday and will belong to someone else tomorrow. The cause of your misery is the illusory happiness that you derive by thinking about the things you own.

- Change is a rule of nature. What you think is death is actually life. Remove mine and yours, small and big from your mind. Then everything is yours, and you are for everyone.

- This body does not belong to you, and neither do you belong to this body. This body is made of elements found in nature and will go back into nature.

- Whatever you do, do it with a sense of detachment without owning and then you will always feel free and happy.

Note: Adapted from Eastern philosophy from India as described in *Bhagvad Gita,* the Holy Scripture of Hindus.

* * * * *

Worksheet 6.1
Taylor Manifest Anxiety Scale

Indicate whether each item is true or false for you.

____ 1. I do not tire quickly.

____ 2. I am troubled by attacks of nausea.

____ 3. I believe I am no more nervous than most others.

____ 4. I have very few headaches.

____ 5. I work under a great deal of tension.

____ 6. I cannot keep my mind on one thing.

____ 7. I worry over money and business.

____ 8. I frequently notice that my hand shakes when I try to do something.

____ 9. I blush no more often than others.

____ 10. I have diarrhea once a month or more.

____ 11. I worry quite a bit over possible misfortunes.

____ 12. I practically never blush.

____ 13. I am often afraid that I am going to blush.

____ 14. I have nightmares every few nights.

____ 15. My hands and feet are usually warm enough.

____ 16. I sweat very easily even on cool days.

____ 17. Sometimes when embarrassed, I break out in a sweat, which annoys me greatly.

____ 18. I hardly ever notice my heart pounding, and I am seldom short of breath.

____ 19. I feel hungry almost all the time.

Worksheet 6.1 Taylor Manifest Anxiety Scale (cont'd)

____ 20. I am very seldom troubled by constipation.

____ 21. I have a great deal of stomach trouble.

____ 22. I have had periods in which I lost sleep over worry.

____ 23. My sleep is fitful and disturbed.

____ 24. I dream frequently about things that are best kept to myself.

____ 25. I am easily embarrassed.

____ 26. I am more sensitive than most other people.

____ 27. I frequently find myself worrying about something.

____ 28. I wish I could be as happy as others seem to be.

____ 29. I am usually calm and not easily upset.

____ 30. I cry easily.

____ 31. I feel anxiety about something or someone almost all the time.

____ 32. I am happy most of the time.

____ 33. It makes me nervous to have to wait.

____ 34. I have periods of such great restlessness that I cannot sit long in a chair.

____ 35. Sometimes I become so excited that I find it hard to get to sleep.

____ 36. I have sometimes felt that difficulties were piling up so high that I could not overcome them.

____ 37. I must admit that I have at times been worried beyond reason over something that really did not matter.

____ 38. I have very few fears compared to my friends.

____ 39. I have been afraid of things or people that I know could not hurt me.

Worksheet 6.1 Taylor Manifest Anxiety Scale (cont'd)

____ 40. I certainly feel useless at times.

____ 41. I find it hard to keep my mind on a task or job.

____ 42. I am usually self-conscious.

____ 43. I am inclined to take things hard.

____ 44. I am a high-strung person.

____ 45. Life is a strain for me much of the time.

____ 46. At times I think I am no good at all.

____ 47. I am certainly lacking in self-confidence.

____ 48. I sometimes feel that I am about to go to pieces.

____ 49. I shrink from facing a crisis or difficulty.

____ 50. I am entirely self-confident.

Note: From "A personality scale of manifest anxiety" by J. A. Taylor, 1953, *Journal of Abnormal and Social Psychology, 48,* 285–290. Copyright 1953 by Journal of Abnormal and Social Psychology. Material under public domain.

FEEDBACK ON WORKSHEET 6.1

To score on this scale give yourself one point for each of the following responses:

1. False	11. True	21. True	31. True	41. True
2. True	12. False	22. True	32. False	42. True
3. False	13. True	23. True	33. True	43. True
4. False	14. True	24. True	34. True	44. True
5. True	15. False	25. True	35. True	45. True
6. True	16. True	26. True	36. True	46. True
7. True	17. True	27. True	37. True	47. True
8. True	18. False	28. True	38. False	48. True
9. False	19. True	29. False	39. True	49. True
10. True	20. False	30. True	40. True	50. False

The average score on this scale is approximately 19. If you scored below that, you feel less anxious than the average person, and if you scored above that, you feel more anxious than the average person. If you scored over 35 on this scale, then your anxiety levels are very high and you need to curb this tendency.

* * * * *

The Taylor Manifest Anxiety Scale measures what is known as *trait anxiety.* If your score is over 35 in the Taylor scale, it indicates that your anxiety is evidencing itself in physical and/or psychological symptoms and warrants serious attention (Allen & Hyde, 1980). Therefore, it is necessary for you to master the techniques presented in this chapter. The other type of anxiety is *state anxiety,* which is temporary in nature and is usually associated with a stimulus. This state anxiety is situation specific. The techniques presented in this chapter when practiced over a long time will help in coping with state anxiety also.

Coping Mechanisms

I. Method Based on Rational Emotive Therapy (Dryden & DiGiuseppe, 1990; Ellis, 1971, 1975a, 1975b, 1990; Ellis & Grieger, 1977; Ellis & Harper, 1961; Walen, DiGiuseppe, & Wessler, 1980).

We are constantly engaging in self-talk, that is, the internal thought language by way of which we describe and interpret the world around us. If the beliefs of our self-talk are in consonance with reality, then we function well. If the beliefs are irrational and untrue, then they cause stress and emotional disturbance. Ellis's method of Rational Emotive Therapy (RET) essentially challenges or refutes this very irrational thinking.

In RET, to be rational, we must be (a) practical, (b) logical, (c) objective, and (d) reality-based. On this basis, *rationality* is an attribute that helps us to achieve our basic goals and purposes in life, to be logical, and to be consistently aware of reality. On the other hand, *irrationality* prevents us from achieving our basic goals and purposes, is illogical (especially dogmatic), and is inconsistent with reality. Based upon Rational Emotive Therapy, some of the classical irrational ideas are depicted in Thoughts for Reflection 6.2.

Thoughts for Reflection 6.2
Rational Emotive Therapy's 11 Irrational Ideas

1. The idea that it is a dire necessity to be loved or approved by virtually every other significant person.
2. The idea that one should be thoroughly competent, adequate, and achieving in all possible respects if one is to consider oneself worthwhile.
3. The idea that certain people are bad, wicked, or villainous and that they should be severely punished and blamed for their villainy.
4. The idea it is awful and catastrophic when things are not the way one would very much like them to be.
5. The idea that human unhappiness is externally controlled, and that people have no ability to control their unhappiness.
6. The idea that something is or may be dangerous or fearsome, one should be concerned about it, and should keep dwelling on the possibility of its occurring.
7. The idea that it is easier to avoid than to face certain life difficulties and self-responsibilities.
8. The idea that one's past history is an all-important determiner of one's present behavior and that because something once strongly affected one's life, it should indefinitely have a similar effect.
9. The idea that one should be dependent on others and need someone stronger than oneself on whom to rely.
10. The idea that one should become quite upset over other people's problems.
11. The idea that there is invariably a right, precise, and perfect solution to human problems, and that it is catastrophic if this perfect solution is not found.

Note: From *RET handbook of rational emotive therapy* by A. Ellis and R. Grieger, 1977, New York: Springer Publishing Company. Copyright 1977 Springer Publishing Company, Inc., New York 10012. Used by permission.

* * * * *

The method based upon RET is popularly known as the ABCDE technique and consists of five steps:

A. *Activating System.* The activating system may be either external or internal events that we face. It also comprises inferences or interpretations about events around us.

B. *Belief System.* The belief system consists of evaluative ideas or constructed views about the world around us. These ideas may either be rigid or flexible. When these beliefs become rigid, they are usually irrational and take the form of "musts," "shoulds," "have to's," "got to's," and so on. These beliefs express themselves as

- "Awfulizing," that is, classifying any situation as 100 percent bad
- "I can't stand it," that is, low frustration tolerance
- "Damnation," that is, being excessively critical of self, others, and/or life conditions
- "Always-and-never thinking," that is, usage of extreme terms

When our beliefs are flexible, they are rational. These beliefs often take the form of desires, wishes, wants, and preferences. These rational beliefs express themselves as

- Moderate evaluations of badness, for example, "It is bad, but it is not terrible."
- Statements of toleration, for example, "I don't like it, but I can bear it."
- Acceptance of fallibility, for example, "I was wrong."
- Avoidance of extremes, for example, "Often I do well." (Instead of "I always do well.")

C. *Consequences.* Our beliefs have emotional and behavioral consequences. If our beliefs about negative activating events are rigid and irrational, then they result in disturbance and are termed inappropriate negative consequences. However, if our beliefs about negative activating events are flexible and rational, then they do not result in any disturbance and are termed appropriate negative consequences.

D. *Dispute Irrational Beliefs.* Disputing irrational beliefs is the key component needed in order for this method to be effective. If we dispute the irrational beliefs in our mind, then we can also reduce the negative consequences that result.

E. *Effect.* As a result of disputing the irrational beliefs in our mind, we experience a new and more desirable consequence, which is referred to as the effect in this method. You may now work through these steps using Worksheet 6.2.

Worksheet 6.2
Anxiety Reduction through RET

Seek out a quiet place, and put aside everything else that you have been doing. Now follow the steps outlined below.

***Step 1.* Activating System**

This step entails identifying the stressor. In the following space write down the facts of a recent event at a time when you were upset. Include only objective facts, not conjectures, subjective impressions, or value judgments.

____

____

____

____

***Step 2.* Belief System**

This step entails identifying the rational and irrational beliefs associated with the event. In the following space, write down all your judgments, beliefs, assumptions, perceptions, and worries pertaining to the event of Step 1.

____

____

____

____

***Step 3.* Consequences**

Identify the physical, mental, and behavioral results. Try to present these in the form of a summary word or words, for example, *anger, grief.*

____

____

____

____

Worksheet 6.2 Anxiety Reduction through RET (cont'd)

***Step 4.* Dispute Irrational Beliefs**

a. Select *one* irrational belief at a time.

____

b. Is there any rational support for this idea? Your response needs to be "NO."

c. Assign reasons for this falseness.

____

____

d. What is the worst thing that can happen according to this irrational idea?

____

____

e. What are the good things that can happen if you do not accept this irrational idea?

____

____

***Step 5.* Effect**

Prepare for the worst events that can happen if you accept this irrational belief. Focus on the benefits that can occur if you do not accept this irrational belief. Give autosuggestions (self-talk) to refute this irrational belief. As a consequence of this new thinking, you will experience the positive results. Proceed in a similar fashion with other irrational ideas, and practice this technique regularly.

* * * * *

II. Method Based on Simplified Kundalini Yoga (SKY) (Maharishi, 1989).

The Simplified Kundalini Yoga (SKY) method, derived from Indian philosophy, is based on the principles of introspection as advocated by Yogiraj Vethathiri Maharishi, a contemporary philosopher and teacher from India who has formed the World Community Service Center, which has branches all over the world (see Chapter 3). This method entails the following steps:

Step 1. We need to seek a quiet place, have available at least one-half hour of uninterrupted time, and have a sheet of paper and pencil with us.

Step 2. This step involves thinking, contemplating, and compiling a list of all the worries that are bothering us at the present time.

Step 3. In this step we classify the worries into four types:

a. *Worries That Should Be Faced.* For example, a child is born with a birth defect (congenital anomaly). Despite all the best efforts, he or she cannot be cured by any medicine or other means. How can we solve this worry? What is the use of brooding over such a worry? In order to manage such worries, we need to resolve to be aware that there is no use worrying over things over which we have no control. Make your mind firm and abide by this resolution. In this category worries like chronic diseases, loss of property, and death will be listed.

b. *Worries to Be Solved Immediately.* Some worries have to be dealt with immediately and boldly. For example, one such worry is about general illness. It can be managed immediately by resorting to proper medication, diet, and lifestyle changes.

Similarly, such worries can arise out of differences of opinion in the family. We cannot disown our families; therefore, these worries need to be managed by mutual discussion without any delay. Other worries about poverty and debts can be managed by hard work, perseverance, and economy in spending.

c. *Worries That May Be Postponed.* For example, consider a person who has reached an age suitable for marriage and is not able to find the right partner. For tackling such a worry, he or she has to keep on trying patiently and allow time to take its course. Therefore, action on such a worry can be postponed.

d. *Worries to Be Ignored.* For example, your boss has a habit of constantly nagging you with his/her outmoded ideas and notions. The best thing to do in such a situation would be to quietly keep on doing your best, unmindful of the purposeless advice given to you. In this category, worries arising out of differences of opinion, jealousy, and the like will be listed.

Step 4. Having classified all our worries into four types, the total number of worries to be tackled at the present time will be reduced. An unnecessary burden on our mind will be eased. Do not think that there will be no more worries in the future or that these worries will completely cease to exist. After one worry is resolved, another one will "spring up." After we climb one mountain, another peak will come into our vision to be conquered. But what we can do now is work in a planned way to reduce our worries. Worksheet 6.3 helps you to classify your worries according to this method in order to lessen the burden on your mind.

Worksheet 6.3
Anxiety Reduction through SKY

Seek out a quiet place for at least one-half hour of contemplation. Think about and compile your worries into the following categories:

Worries to Be Faced	***Worries to Be Solved Immediately***	***Worries to Be Postponed***	***Worries to Be Ignored***

Note: From *Yoga for modern age* (3rd ed.) by Y. V. Maharishi, 1989, Madras, India: Vethathiri Publications. Copyright 1989 by Y. V. Maharishi. Reprinted by permission.

FEEDBACK ON WORKSHEET 6.3

Classification of the worries bothering your mind into the four categories must have resulted in reducing the total number of worries to be tackled at the *present* time. This will reduce an unnecessary burden on your mind. In this way whenever your mind is flooded with a number of worries and problems, you can sit down and practice this technique to reduce the total number of worries at any time. This is a useful and effective approach that conserves energy you can use for other productive activities.

* * * * *

III. Method Based on Gestalt Therapy (Corey, 1991; Corsini, 1984; Perls, 1969)

Gestalt is a German word meaning "whole" or "configuration" (Simkin, 1976). As one psychological dictionary puts it, Gestalt is "an integration of the whole as contrasted with summation of parts" (Warren, 1934). The originator of Gestalt therapy, Fredrick S. Perls, drew an analogy of the concept of this theory with an organism that always works as a whole. Organisms are not a summation of parts but a coordination of organ systems or other components (Perls, 1969). Gestalt therapy emphasizes the unity of self-awareness behavior and experience. The goal of Gestalt therapy is to help us get in touch with reality and focus on the "now." It implicitly asks individuals to accept that they will be more comfortable and effective in their lives in the long run if they are fully aware of what they are doing from moment to moment and accept responsibility for their behaviors. By discovering *what is* rather than what should be or what could have been, or the ideal of what should be or may be, the person learns to trust himself or herself. A Gestalt prayer summarizes this philosophy (Perls, 1969):

I do my thing, and you do your thing.
I am not in this world to live up to your expectations
And you are not in this world to live up to mine.
You are you, and I am I,
And if by chance we find each other, it's beautiful.
If not, it can't be helped.

A modified process based on the principles of this Gestalt therapy is provided in Worksheet 6.4 for you to practice.

Worksheet 6.4
Coping with Anxiety Based on Gestalt Therapy

Go through the following steps, and write down your responses wherever needed:

Step 1. Seek out a quiet place and focus your awareness on your thinking.

Step 2. Write down the thoughts that are coming into your mind, and at the same time be consciously aware of your body movements, if any.

Thoughts:

____

____

____

____

____

____

____

____

____

____

____

____

____

____

____

____

____

____

Worksheet 6.4 Coping with Anxiety Based on Gestalt Therapy (cont'd)

Body movements/sensations during thoughts:

____

____

____

____

____

Step 3. List the painful thoughts that you do not want to come into your mind.

____

____

____

____

____

Step 4. Experience the pain associated with your thoughts with awareness rather than alleviating it. If painful thoughts become too overbearing, then you should stop and relax.

FEEDBACK ON WORKSHEET 6.4

Try to establish consonance between your thoughts and your body movements. If you are not able to derive any inferences, do not worry—just proceed. Practice this awareness-building exercise and *always focus on now,* that is, on the thoughts that are arising at this moment in time. If painful thoughts become too overbearing, then you should stop and relax. This method can be practiced individually or in groups. With regular practice your skills in coping with anxiety will increase.

* * * * *

IV. Systematic Desensitization

The systematic densensitization technique was first described by Joseph Wolpe (1958, 1973) and involves imagining or experiencing an anxiety-provoking scene while practicing a response incompatible with anxiety (such as relaxation). This concept is also utilized in the field of medicine for treating allergies. The allergic patient is exposed to very small doses of allergen that are gradually increased until the body learns to accept the allergen. In coping with anxiety, the basic method entails slow and steady adjustments to small components of any problem. Each small step is considered one at a time, and relaxation is practiced alongside to counteract the adverse response. This technique involves developing a fear hierarchy, which is a sequence of small steps that lead to the anxiety-provoking event. Consider an example. Suppose we are students and we have test anxiety. Our fear hierarchy would be as follows:

1. Enrolling for the course
2. Going to the classes
3. Completing the assignments
4. Studying the textbook
5. Studying additional materials
6. Reviewing the text
7. Preparing for examinations
8. Going to the examination
9. Waiting before the examination
10. Taking the examination
11. Waiting for the results of the examination
12. Obtaining the results

Most of the test anxiety is tied into the *expectations* of obtaining a good result, and therefore we have included that dimension in the fear hierarchy. Similarly we can construct a fear hierarchy for any fear that causes us anxiety. This procedure has been described systematically in a step-by-step fashion in Worksheet 6.5 for you to practice.

Worksheet 6.5
Systematic Desensitization

You should proceed according to the following steps:

Step 1. Seek a quiet, comfortable, and peaceful place. Select a relaxation technique described in Chapter 3 and relax. Write down the name of this technique on the line:

____

Print the word "relax" on the next line:

____

Step 2. Now you should develop a fear hierarchy for the fear that causes you anxiety. Write down all the *small steps* leading to that fear. You should try to come up with a minimum of 10 steps.

Fear: ____

Hierarchy:

a. ____

b. ____

c. ____

d. ____

e. ____

f. ____

g. ____

h. ____

i. ____

j. ____

Worksheet 6.5 Systematic Desensitization (cont'd)

Step 3. Relax.

Step 4. Imagine the first item in the fear-hierarchy list for one to five seconds. Gradually increase the thinking time to about a minute.

Step 5. Relax.

Step 6. Repeat Step 4 on the next item. If you have difficulty with any item, break it down further into smaller steps and approach it gradually in your mind. You need to reassure yourself that there is nothing to fear.

FEEDBACK ON WORKSHEET 6.5

With regular practice of this technique, you will be able to get over your fear and reduce anxiety when you encounter that event. In this way you will be able to strengthen your mind and not be bogged down by small fears.

* * * * *

Box 6.1 Emotional Intelligence

In recent years a school of thought in psychological research has emerged that emphasizes that the role of emotional maturity is as important as or even more important than intelligence for success in academics and life. Partly, this concept has emerged because, while intelligence quotient (IQ) does predict academic achievement and occupational status, it is able to account for only 10–20 percent of the personal variation in these areas. The other developments that have contributed to greater interest in this line of thought include a recent popular book by Daniel Goleman (1995) on the subject, coverage of this concept in some popular television talk shows, and some empirical research (Mayer & Salovey, 1997). Emotional intelligence has been defined as the ability to use emotions to solve problems. The primary components of emotional intelligence that have been identified are these (Goleman, 1995):

1. *Self-awareness* involves knowing ones emotions, recognizing feelings as they occur, and discriminating between them.
2. *Mood management* entails handling feelings so that they become relevant to the current situation and one reacts appropriately.
3. *Self-motivation* includes "gathering up" one's feelings and directing oneself toward a goal, despite self-doubt, inertia, and impulsiveness.
4. *Empathy* is the ability to recognize feelings in others and tune into their verbal and nonverbal cues.
5. *Managing relationships* requires handling interpersonal interaction, conflict resolution, and negotiations.

Research continues in refining these constructs, measuring these attributes, and ascertaining their contribution and applicability in various facets of life. For the reader in stress management, it would be worthwhile to explore the role of each of these dimensions for anxiety reduction in particular. The major shift required for transcribing this concept is the focus on one's emotions rather than cognitive abilities. While there is indeed an overlap between cognition (thinking) and emotions, perhaps a greater awareness of the latter can enhance one's effectiveness. In simple terms, the following five steps would be helpful in this endeavor:

- Recognizing feelings in oneself
- Recognizing feelings in others
- Caring for others' feelings
- Regulating feelings in oneself
- Harnessing feelings to improving relationships

* * * * *

You should practice all the techniques described in this chapter and find the one that is best for you. Keep practicing that technique to obtain the best results. You may want to change from one technique to another over time, or you may want to practice the same technique. The approach will vary from one person to another.

Stress Management Principle 6

Wipe out anxiety before it wipes you out.

Summary Points

- Anxiety arises out of inefficiency and fear.
- Excessive anxiety is associated with Generalized Anxiety Disorder and Panic Disorder.
- The Taylor Manifest Anxiety Scale measures trait anxiety.
- The Rational Emotive Therapy (RET)–based ABCDE technique described by Albert Ellis consists of five steps: identifying the activating system, identifying the belief system, identifying the consequences, disputing irrational beliefs, and visualizing the effects.
- Coping with anxiety using Simplified Kundalini Yoga as described by Yogiraj Vethathiri Maharishi consists of classifying worries into those to be faced, those to be solved immediately, those to be postponed, and those to be ignored.
- Coping with anxiety using Gestalt therapy described by Fredrick Perls helps us to focus on the "now," discovering "what is reality," and bearing the pain, if any.
- Systematic desensitization described by Joseph Wolpe involves analyzing any anxiety-provoking situation in terms of smaller steps and counteracting those steps at each stage by practicing relaxation.

References and Further Readings

Allen, R. J., & Hyde, D. (1980). *Investigations in stress control.* Minneapolis: Burgess.

Corey, G. (1991). *Theory and practice of counseling and psychotherapy.* Pacific Grove, CA: Brooks/Cole.

Corsini, R. J., & Wedding, D. (1995). *Current psychotherapies* (5th ed.). Itasca, IL: Peacock.

Diagnostic and statistical manual of mental disorders (4th ed.). (DSM IV). (1994). Washington, DC: American Psychiatric Association.

Dryden, W., & DiGiuseppe, R. (1990). *A primer on rational emotive therapy.* Champaign, IL: Research Press.

Ellis, A. (1971). *Growth through reason.* Palo Alto, CA: Science & Behavior.

Ellis, A. (1975a). *A new guide to rational living.* North Hollywood, CA: Wilshire.

Ellis, A. (1975b). *How to live with a neurotic at home and at work* (rev. ed.). North Hollywood, CA: Wilshire.

Ellis, A. (1990). *How to stubbornly refuse to make yourself miserable about anything—yes anything.* New York: Carol.

Ellis, A., & Grieger, R. (1977). *RET handbook of rational emotive therapy.* New York: Springer.

Ellis, A., & Harper, R. (1961). *A guide to rational living.* North Hollywood, CA: Wilshire.

Goleman, D. (1995). *Emotional intelligence: Why it can matter more than IQ for character, health and lifelong achievement.* New York: Bantam.

Greenberg, J. S. (1999). *Comprehensive stress management* (6th ed.). Boston: William C. Brown/McGraw-Hill.

Maharishi, Y. V. (1989). *Yoga for modern age* (3rd ed.). Madras, India: Vethathiri.

Mayer, J. D., & Salovey, P. (1997). What is emotional intelligence? In P. Salovey & D. Sluyter (eds.), *Emotional development, emotional literacy and emotional intelligence.* New York: Basic Books.

Perls, F. S. (1969). *Gestalt therapy verbatim.* Moab, UT: Real People Press.

Regier, D. A., Boyd, J. H., Burke, J. D., Jr., et al. (1988). One month prevalence of mental disorders in the United States: Based on five epidemiological catchment area sites. *Archives of General Psychiatry, 45,* 977–986.

Shader, R. I., & Greenblatt, D. J. (1993). Use of benzodiazepines in anxiety disorders. *New England Journal of Medicine, 328,* 1398–1405.

Simkin, J. S. (1976). *Gestalt therapy: Mini lectures.* Millbrae, CA: Celestial Arts.

Taylor, J. A. (1953). A personality scale of manifest anxiety. *Journal of Abnormal and Social Psychology, 48,* 285–290.

Walen, S. R., DiGiuseppe, R., & Wessler, R. L. (1980). *A practitioner's guide to rational emotive therapy.* New York: Oxford University Press.

Warren, H. D. (1934). *Dictionary of Psychology.* New York: Houghton Mifflin.

Wolpe, J. (1958). *Psychotherapy by reciprocal inhibition.* Stanford, CA: Stanford University Press.

Wolpe, J. (1973). *The practice of behavior therapy* (2nd ed.). New York: Pergamon.

CHAPTER 7

Balanced Diet and Appropriate Eating

Bien haya el que inventó el sueño,
capa que cubre todos los humanos pensamientos,
manjar que quita la hambre,
agua que ahuyenta la sed,
fuego que calienta el frio,
frio que templa el ardor, y, finalmente,
moneda general conque todas las cosas se compran,
balanza y peso que iguala al pastor con el rey
y al simple con el discreto.

[Blessings on him who invented sleep,
the mantle that covers all human thoughts,
the food that satisfies hunger,
the drink that slakes thirst,
the fire that warms cold,
the cold that moderates heat, and, lastly,
the common currency that buys all things,
the balance and weight that equalizes the shepherd
and the king
the simpleton and the sage.]

—*Miguel de Cervantes*

Importance of Balanced Diet and Appropriate Eating

Belloc and Breslow (1972), after surveying nearly 7000 individuals, identified seven behaviors related to the maintenance of personal health:

1. Sleeping seven to eight hours daily
2. Eating breakfast almost daily
3. Consuming planned snacks
4. Being at or near prescribed weight (gender and height specific)
5. Never smoking cigarettes

6. Moderate or no use of alcohol
7. Regular physical activity

While the exact role and mechanism of each of these factors has not been completely understood, it has generally been accepted that all these factors contribute significantly toward maintaining health and longevity. In this chapter we shall primarily be focusing on diet and related eating behaviors. The importance of eating nutritious meals appropriately plays a significant role in healthy living, helps combat daily stress, and also reduces undue stress. Though the relationship between diet and stress has not been studied extensively (Greenberg, 1999), the importance of eating a balanced diet to maintain health and reduce stress cannot be ruled out (Girdano, Everly, & Dusek, 1997). Consumption of a healthy balanced diet enhances our coping abilities against various stressors and stressful events. When our meals consist of all the ingredients of a balanced diet, then our body has sufficient energy to cope with stress. A balanced diet also provides enough reserves to manage stress. Irregular eating of meals, eating improper food (that is, undercooked or overcooked, too spicy or too bland, consisting of only one category of food, stale, unpalatable, and so on), undereating, or overeating unduly taxes the body and is a potential source of stress in itself. If we eat these meals after sufficient appetite has set in, and do not indulge in overeating, then the body is saved from undue stress and associated negative consequences. However, undereating also creates stress for the body because not enough energy is available to perform daily activities. Therefore, the key lies in maintaining a *balance* of quantity and quality of food and regularity in eating.

Enhancing Awareness about Our Dietary Patterns

How well do we eat? Is our diet balanced? Do we eat our meals regularly? These are some of the questions that we may not be able to answer impromptu. The reason is that most of us have become quite used to eating food daily. We seldom take time to think about what we eat and how we eat. We have taken eating for granted. We need to become aware about our diet and eating patterns and consider a change. This awareness about our diet and eating patterns is a central and important step in effecting a change in our behavior. Therefore, before you proceed any further, become more aware of your own dietary habits and patterns with the help of Worksheet 7.1.

Worksheet 7.1
Enhancing Awareness about Diet and Eating

Think about the following items and respond to them in order to obtain feedback regarding your dietary habits and patterns:

1. Height ___________
2. Weight ___________
3. What weight is appropriate for me? ___________
4. When was the last time that I recorded my weight? ___________
5. How often do I record my weight?

   ________ Daily

   ________ Weekly

   ________ Fortnightly

   ________ Monthly

   ________ Bimonthly

   ________ Quarterly

   ________ Yearly

   ________ Whenever I feel like it

   ________ Sometimes, irregularly

   ________ Never

6. Do I eat breakfast?

   ________ Regularly every day

   ________ Occasionally

   ________ Never

7. Do I eat between meals?

   ________ Always

   ________ Occasionally

   ________ Never

Worksheet 7.1 Enhancing Awareness about Diet and Eating (cont'd)

8. Do I drink coffee, tea or colas?

_______ Every day What type? ____________________

How much? ____________________

_______ Occasionally What type? ____________________

How much? ____________________

_______ Never

9. Do I smoke tobacco products?

_______ Every day What type? ____________________

How much? ____________________

_______ Occasionally What type? ____________________

How much? ____________________

_______ Never

10. Do I drink alcoholic beverages?

_______ Every day What type? ____________________

How much? ____________________

_______ Occasionally What type? ____________________

How much? ____________________

_______ Never

11. Do I take any illegal drugs?

_______ Yes What type? ____________________

How much? ____________________

_______ No

12. Do I eat the following food items at least once per day? (Put a check mark next to each one that applies.)

_______ Canned foods

_______ Processed cheese

Worksheet 7.1 Enhancing Awareness about Diet and Eating (cont'd)

_______ Seasonings

_______ Sausage/ham/ bacon (red meat)

_______ Chips (potato/corn/tortilla)

_______ Table salt

_______ Pizza

_______ "Fast foods"

13. How often do I eat chocolate?

_______ Never

_______ Rarely

_______ Often

_______ Sometimes

_______ Daily

14. What is my level of sugar consumption (namely, candy)?

_______ Excessive

_______ Moderate

_______ Adequate

_______ Less than normal

FEEDBACK ON WORKSHEET 7.1

Items 1–3. Ideal weight depends upon gender, height, and build. Information about ideal weight based upon height, body frame, and gender is depicted in Table 7.1. In order to check your ideal weight, you first need to assess your build. Then find out your height and look for the range of your weight in the table.

FEEDBACK ON WORKSHEET 7.1 (cont'd)

Table 7.1 Weight Chart

MEN

Acceptable Weight (pounds, without clothing)

Height	*Small Frame*	*Medium Frame*	*Large Frame*
5′1″	123–129	126–136	133–145
5′2″	125–131	128–138	135–148
5′3″	127–133	130–140	137–151
5′4″	129–135	132–143	139–155
5′5″	131–137	134–146	141–159
5′6″	133–140	137–149	144–163
5′7″	135–143	140–152	147–167
5′8″	137–146	143–155	150–171
5′9″	139–149	146–158	153–175
5′10″	141–152	149–161	156–179
5′11″	144–155	152–165	159–183
6′0″	147–159	155–169	163–187
6′1″	150–163	159–173	167–192
6′2″	153–167	162–177	171–197
6′3″	157–171	166–182	176–202

WOMEN

Acceptable Weight (pounds, without clothing)

Height	*Small Frame*	*Medium Frame*	*Large Frame*
4′9″	99–108	106–118	115–128
4′10″	100–110	108–120	117–131
4′11″	101–112	110–123	119–134
5′0″	103–115	112–126	122–137
5′1″	105–118	115–129	125–140
5′2″	108–121	118–132	128–144
5′3″	111–124	121–135	131–148
5′4″	114–127	124–138	134–152
5′5″	117–130	127–141	137–156
5′6″	120–133	130–144	140–160
5′7″	123–136	133–147	143–164
5′8″	126–139	136–150	146–167
5′9″	129–142	139–153	149–170
5′10″	132–145	142–156	152–173
5′11″	135–148	145–159	155–176

Note: From *The American Medical Association family medical guide,* p. 28, by the American Medical Association. Copyright © 1982 by the American Medical Association. Reprinted by permission of Random House, Inc.

FEEDBACK ON WORKSHEET 7.1 (cont'd)

Items 4–5. You need to maintain your weight based upon the ideal range for your height, body frame, and gender. Therefore, you should record your weight regularly. A written record provides a chronological baseline to compare and make changes as necessary. However, you should not be fanatical about recording weights too often because weight changes are slow to occur. It is good to record weight fortnightly or monthly.

Item 6. Research indicates that hypoglycemia or low blood sugar predisposes an individual to stress. Symptoms of hypoglycemia may include anxiety, headache, dizziness, trembling, and increased cardiac activity (Girdano, Everly, & Dusek, 1997). The best way to avoid stress associated with hypoglycemia, for a normal person, is to eat a balanced breakfast every day.

Item 7. Eating continuously between meals unduly activates the digestive system, leading to a release of various chemicals and by-products that may add to the stress getting built up. This self-induced stress can be controlled by planning to consume food more appropriately.

Item 8. Coffee, tea, and colas have *caffeine,* which is identified as a sympathomimetic agent or a pseudostressor. When consumed, they trigger a stress response in the body. A six-ounce cup of coffee (*Coffea arabica*) contains about 108 milligrams of caffeine; tea (*Camelia sinensis*) contains 90 mg/cup. Various cola beverages contain 50–60 mg/12 oz., and a bar of chocolate (1 oz.) about 20 mg (Girdano, Everly, Dusek, 1997).

Item 9. Nicotine found in tobacco is also a sympathomimetic agent and produces a stress response in the body. Tobacco smoke also contains various other harmful products such as tar and carbon monoxide that can lead to bronchitis, lung cancer, and other diseases.

Item 10. Alcohol is a central nervous system inhibitor, although it may appear to reduce stress. However, stress is known to be tied to alcohol addiction (Schlaadt, 1992). There are approximately 10 to 13 million alcoholics in the United States and more than 7 million alcohol abusers. Alcohol abuse is at the root of impaired job performance, child abuse, spouse abuse, accidental injuries, and medical disorders (*Seventh Special Report to the U.S. Congress on Alcohol and Health,* 1990).

Item 11. Illegal drugs may be grouped into *five categories: stimulants,* like cocaine; marijuana and its derivatives; *depressants,* such as the opiates; *psychedelics; deliriants;* and "*designer drugs*" (Ray & Ksir, 1999). These drugs do not relieve stress. In fact they add to the stress response in the long run. Adopting these negative mechanisms for temporary relief of stress can be extremely hazardous and ruin our physical, mental, and social well-being.

FEEDBACK ON WORKSHEET 7.1 (cont'd)

Item 12. Fast foods and other products mentioned in the list are rich in *sodium* content. Sodium is a mineral responsible for regulating water balance in the body. The United States Recommended Dietary Allowances suggest no more than 2400 milligrams of sodium per day. If the products that you have checked are high in sodium, it is important to restrict their usage. A good nutritious diet provides the necessary sodium, and excessive sodium may contribute to an increase in blood pressure and stress (Greenberg, 1999).

Item 13. Chocolate contains *caffeine* and *sugar.* Caffeine, as explained earlier, is a pseudostressor or a sympathomimetic agent. It induces a response in the body that is akin to the stress response. Excess sugar provides the body with unused energy, and this usually leads to the accumulation of harmful by-products. Both these products therefore add to our stress and need to be avoided.

Item 14. Excessive sugar, as has been explained, leaves excess unused energy in the body. This does not relieve stress, but in fact adds to stress levels. Moreover, consuming large quantities of sugar over a long period may contribute to weight gain and various diseases directly or indirectly, such as diabetes mellitus. Therefore, it is best to regulate the intake of sugar in our diets.

* * * * *

Categories of Food Items

Let us briefly understand the various types of food items and what they do to our body. The various food items can be classified, from a nutrition point of view, into the following six categories:

1. *Carbohydrates:* Carbohydrate is a word of chemistry. Chemically, the word "carbohydrate" is derived from "carbo" implying carbon and "hydrate" implying hydrogen and oxygen. That is, these compounds are constituted of varying proportions of carbon, hydrogen, and oxygen. Food items rich in carbohydrates include sugars, bread (wheat flour), the fibrous lining of fruits and vegetables, cereals, rice, pasta (wheat flour), roots and tubers, and so on. These food items when consumed and digested provide the body with *energy.* This energy helps the body perform its daily activities. They also provide the diet with fiber, which adds to the bulk and facilitates easy elimination from the bowel. It is important to consume these vital categories of food products in *moderation.* If too little carbohydrate is consumed, then the body does not get enough energy to perform daily tasks. If it is ingested in excess, the body tends to convert and store these products for future use. If this excess carbohydrate persists for a long time and is at the cost of other vital food items, then fat deposition and other health-related problems occur. Further, if our diet solely consists of carbohydrates, then the body is deprived of other vital categories of food items and the body is weakened, especially in coping with long-term demands of stress. Thus the importance of using moderation and combining this category with other food categories cannot be overemphasized. Determining the correct amount of carbohydrates to be consumed is dependent upon many factors including the amount of daily activity, type of activities, body constitution, and so on. As a general rule, 6-11 servings of grain products are recommended per day by the U.S. Department of Agriculture (see Figure 7.1). If our activity levels are more sedentary in nature or if our body constitution is smaller, we may stick to the lower limit of the prescribed range for observing moderation. Use of sugars per se needs to be curtailed. Thoughts for Reflection 7.1 provides some suggestions.

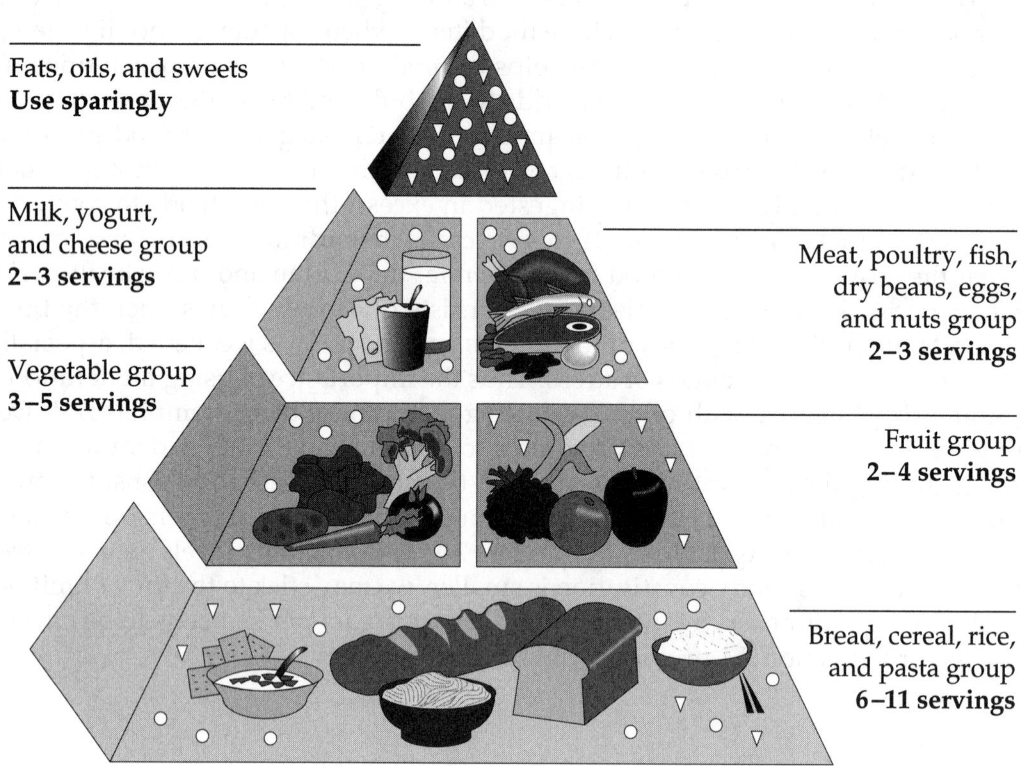

Figure 7.1 Food Pyramid

Note: From U.S. Department of Agriculture

Thoughts for Reflection 7.1
Using Sugars in Moderation—Some Suggestions

At the Supermarket:

- Read ingredient labels. Identify all the added sugars in a product. Select items lower in added sugars when possible.
- Buy fresh fruits or fruits packed in water or juice, rather than those in light or heavy syrup.
- Buy fewer foods that are high in sugars such as soft drinks, fruit-flavored punches, and sweet desserts. Be aware that some low-fat desserts may be very high in sugars.

In the Kitchen:

- Reduce the sugars in foods you prepare at home. Try new recipes or make your own. Start by reducing sugars gradually until you have decreased them by one-third or more.
- Experiment with spices such as cinnamon, cardamom, coriander, nutmeg, ginger, and mace to enhance the sweet flavor of foods. Spiced foods will taste sweeter if warmed.
- When possible, use home-prepared items (made with less sugar) instead of commercially prepared ones that are higher in sugar.

At the Table:

- Use less of all sugars including white and brown sugars, honey, molasses, syrups, jams, and jellies.
- Choose fewer foods that are high in added sugars such as prepared baked goods, candies, and sweet desserts.
- Reach for fresh fruit instead of something sweetened with additional sugars for dessert or a snack.
- Add less sugar to foods—coffee, tea, cereal, or fruit. Get used to using half as much, then see if you can cut back even more.
- Cut back on the number of sugar-sweetened soft drinks, punches, and ades you drink.

Note: From *Use sugars only in moderation* (p. 5) by United States Department of Agriculture (Human Nutrition Information Service), July 1993, Washington D.C.: U.S. Government Printing Office. Material under public domain.

* * * * *

2. *Proteins:* The word "protein" is derived from the Greek word *proteios* meaning prime or chief. Proteins are in fact the most important constituents of our diet. There are two major sources of dietary proteins: (a) *animal sources:* eggs, milk, meat, fish, and so on, and (b) *plant sources:* lentils, cereals, nuts, beans, and so on. The prime function of protein is *body building.* Proteins are needed for growth, maintenance, and replacement of body cells. They are also required in the production of most hormones and enzymes, which regulate body functioning. In order to combat stress, they are important constituents. If the diet lacks enough proteins, then the body becomes emaciated, and stress-fighting capabilities are also substantially reduced. Extreme environmental or physiological stresses increase nitrogen loss through urine and increase energy expenditure (Cuthberston, 1964). This effect necessitates the need for greater amounts of protein intake. However, if the diet contains excess protein, then it is converted to carbohydrate and stored for future use. If this excess persists, then that is also not good for the body. It may lead to unwanted and unused by-products that are potentially harmful. Some proteins are also responsible for allergic manifestations in many susceptible people. Therefore, *moderation* in intake of proteins is essential. According to U.S. Department of Agriculture, 2–3 servings per day from the milk, yogurt, and cheese group and the meat, poultry, fish, dry beans, eggs, and nuts group are recommended (see Figure 7.1).

3. *Fats:* Fats are sources of energy and are important in helping to carry some vitamins (fat-soluble vitamins). Some fats also form cell membranes and hormones. They also add flavor to foods. Dietary fats are derived from two sources: (a) *animal sources:* butter, lard, and so on, and (b) *plant sources:* various edible oils like sunflower, canola, olive, and so on. Fats should be used *sparingly* in the diet. As explained earlier, small quantities of fat are required by the body for performing some vital functions. However, when taken in excess, they tend to accumulate in the body. Excess deposition of fats leads to obesity, which has been associated as a risk factor for a number of disorders including coronary heart disease, stroke, and so on. Thoughts for Reflection 7.2 provides some suggestions for reducing cholesterol and fats in the diet.

Thoughts for Reflection 7.2
Easy Ways to Cut Fat, Saturated Fat, and Cholesterol in Your Diet

At the Store:

- Choose lean cuts of meat, such as beef round, loin, sirloin, pork loin chops, and roasts.
- Consider fish and poultry as alternatives; they are somewhat lower in saturated fat.
- Buy low-fat versions of dairy products.
- Read the food label and choose foods that are lower in fat, saturated fat, and cholesterol.

In the Kitchen:

- When cooking, replace saturated fats, such as butter and lard, with small amounts of polyunsaturated and monounsaturated fats in vegetable oils such as corn oil, soybean oil, olive oil, peanut oil, or canola oil.
- Broil, roast, bake, steam, or boil foods instead of frying them, or try stir-frying with just a little fat.
- Trim all visible fat from meat before it is cooked.
- Spoon off fat from meat dishes after they are cooked.
- Use skim milk or low-fat milk when making cream sauces, soups, or puddings.
- Substitute low-fat yogurt or whipped low-fat cottage cheese for sour cream and mayonnaise in dips and dressings.
- Substitute two egg whites for each whole egg in recipes for most quick breads, cookies, and cakes. (Cholesterol and fat are in the yolk, not in the white.)
- Try lemon juice, herbs, or spices to season foods instead of butter or margarine.

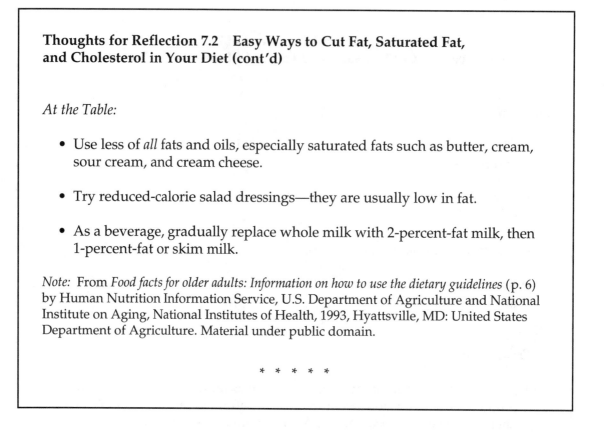

Thoughts for Reflection 7.2 Easy Ways to Cut Fat, Saturated Fat, and Cholesterol in Your Diet (cont'd)

At the Table:

- Use less of *all* fats and oils, especially saturated fats such as butter, cream, sour cream, and cream cheese.
- Try reduced-calorie salad dressings—they are usually low in fat.
- As a beverage, gradually replace whole milk with 2-percent-fat milk, then 1-percent-fat or skim milk.

Note: From *Food facts for older adults: Information on how to use the dietary guidelines* (p. 6) by Human Nutrition Information Service, U.S. Department of Agriculture and National Institute on Aging, National Institutes of Health, 1993, Hyattsville, MD: United States Department of Agriculture. Material under public domain.

* * * * *

4. *Vitamins:* The word "vitamin" is derived from the earlier German word *vitamine* (*vita* meaning life, and *amine* based on the earlier notion that all these substances contained amino acids chemically). Vitamins are substances that are needed by the body in extremely small amounts. Though vitamins do not supply energy directly, they do help in the release of energy from other substances and play an important role in completing many chemical reactions within the body. Vitamins can be broadly classified into two types: (a) *fat soluble:* A, D, E, and K; and (b) *water soluble:* B and C. Some of the key sources of vitamins are depicted in Table 7.2.

Table 7.2 Important Sources of Some Vitamins

Vitamin	*Sources*
A (retinol)	Eggs, whole milk, fish, green leafy vegetables like spinach, cabbage, broccoli; colored vegetables like carrots and pumpkin; fruits like papaya
B_1 (thiamine)	Dried yeast, unmilled cereals, lentils, nuts, and oilseeds
B_2 (riboflavin)	Liver, meat, milk, eggs, germinating lentils, cereals, and vegetables
Niacin	Grain products, milk, eggs (contain tryptophan, which can be converted to niacin)
B_6 (pyridoxine)	Chicken, fish, kidney, liver, pork, eggs, unmilled rice, soybeans, oats, whole wheat products, peanuts, and walnuts
Folic acid	Liver, yeast, leafy vegetables, legumes, and some fruits
B_{12}	Liver, meat, eggs, milk
C (ascorbic acid)	Green and red peppers, collard greens, broccoli, spinach, tomatoes, potatoes, strawberries, oranges, and other citrus fruits
D	Sunlight; fortified milk, fortified margarine, eggs, butter
E	Vegetable oils (soybean, corn, cottonseed, safflower)
K	Green leafy vegetables, milk, meats, eggs, cereals, fruits, and vegetables

If fat-soluble vitamins are consumed in excess, they tend to accumulate in the body. This accumulation is responsible for disorders called hypervitaminosis. There is consensus that these vitamins should not be taken in excess as supplements. Water-soluble vitamins, if taken in excess, are easily excreted out of the system. However, authorities are divided on recommending their excess use. While some believe they cause no harm, others believe that they can be harmful too (for example, taking excess Vitamin C can cause formation of renal stones). We would recommend a balance in taking vitamins. From a stress management point of view, vitamins are essential in optimum quantities for maintaining the body's resistance to stress.

5. *Minerals:* Minerals are also needed in relatively small amounts primarily to make hemoglobin in red blood cells and strengthen bones and teeth. They are also essential to maintain body fluids and chemical reactions in the body. They improve the body's ability to manage stress effectively if taken in *optimum* quantities. Some minerals helpful in combating stress are calcium, iron, zinc, and magnesium. It is also important to reduce the intake of common salt (sodium chloride), which induces retention of body fluids and elicits the stress response. Thoughts for Reflection 7.3 provides some ideas for reducing sodium in your diet.

Thoughts for Reflection 7.3
Some Tips on Reducing Sodium in Your Diet

At the Store:

- Read labels for information on the sodium content.
- Try fresh or plain frozen vegetables and meats instead of those canned or prepared with salt.
- Look for low- or reduced-sodium or "no-salt-added" versions of foods.

In the Kitchen:

- Cook plain rice, pasta, and hot cereals using less salt than the package calls for (try 1/8 teaspoon of salt for two servings). "Instant" rice, pasta, and cereals may contain salt added by the processor.
- Adjust your recipes, gradually cutting down on the amount of salt. If some of the ingredients already contain salt, such as canned soup or vegetables, you may need to add no more salt at all.
- Use herbs and spices as seasonings for vegetables and meats instead of salt.

At the Table:

- Taste your food before you salt it. Does it really need more salt? Try one shake instead of two. Gradually cut down on the amount of salt you use. Your taste will adjust to less salt.

Note: From *Food facts for older adults: Information on how to use the dietary guidelines* (p. 8–9) by Human Nutrition Information Service, U.S. Department of Agriculture and National Institute on Aging, National Institutes of Health, 1993, Hyattsville, MD: United States Department of Agriculture. Material under public domain.

* * * * *

6. *Water:* This extremely important constituent of the diet is most often forgotten. We take water for granted most of the time. In the absence of water life will perish. Water helps to transport all the body nutrients, removes waste products, and regulates body temperature. In order to combat stress effectively, the body needs an adequate supply of water. Water also helps to dilute harmful chemical substances if they are accumulating in the body. Water also helps in excretion of these substances. It is recommended that we drink 8–10 glasses of water every day. This means that water should be consumed at times when one is not even thirsty. It also means that we should not replace water with other beverages, soft drinks, and so on. We have already seen that most beverages, like cola, tea, coffee, and the like, contain caffeine and preservatives that do more harm than good. Hence water is the only constituent of the diet that, for the most part, does no harm to the body and has only beneficial results. We would like to suggest that one consume as much water as possible.

Avoiding Alcohol, Smoking, and Drug Abuse

The issues of alcohol, smoking, and drug abuse are extensive and complex in nature. However, we would like to briefly discuss some points regarding these issues here because many people attempt to find solutions to their stress problems by using, misusing, and abusing chemical substances.

Drinking alcoholic beverages is associated with a number of health problems. Alcoholic beverages supply calories to the body but fail to provide any nutrients. These "empty calories" often lead to malnourishment and decreased capabilities in combating daily stresses. Excessive alcohol use has also been associated as a risk factor with cirrhosis of the liver, inflammation of the pancreas, damage to the brain and heart, and increased risk for a variety of cancers. Alcohol is a central nervous system depressant and therefore decreases reaction time, hampers judgment, and impairs sensory responses. As we have already seen in Chapters 1 and 2, perception of a stressor is central to the effective management of stress. When this perception is distorted by use of alcohol, recuperation from stress is considerably lowered.

Many of us smoke in the belief that we will get relief from stress. However, this is not true. Tobacco smoke contains nicotine, which is a pseudostressor, as we have already seen in Worksheet 7.1. When the body gets habituated to smoking, it requires more nicotine to get the release of normal chemicals, which may falsely give a smoker the feeling of getting relief from stress. This stress is in fact self-inflicted and can be completely avoided. Tobacco smoke has also been associated with a number of health problems including emphysema, bronchitis, lung cancer, and so on. For a pregnant woman, smoking can lead to low birth weight in her child. If one is a smoker, he or she needs to seriously consider quitting. The decision for quitting needs to come from within, then an effective plan can be undertaken.

Most illegal drugs also act on the central nervous system. These drugs can depress the central nervous system, stimulate it, or alter and distort sensory responses. In all cases the net result is poor perception and decreased coping capabilities. Drug abuse also leads to psychological and/or physical dependence. Let us ask ourselves,

- Am I resorting to alcohol use, smoking, or drug use to find answers to my problems?

- Is this the correct decision? *NO*
- How else can I solve my problems?

If alcohol or drug abuse is a problem, we need not let it get out of control and hamper our life. We need to seek professional help at the earliest possible time. We may want to contact a professional counselor, our family physician, or a support organization like Alcoholics Anonymous (AA). The local address of Alcoholics Anonymous can be found in our telephone book.

Box 7.1 Caffeine: What It Is and How Much Is Found in Popular Drinks

Chemically, caffeine is an alkaloid. There are numerous compounds called alkaloids, among them are the methylxanthines, with three well-known compounds: theophylline (found in tea), theobromine (found in cocoa bean), and caffeine. Caffeine is primarily found in coffee, tea, cola nuts, maté, and guarana, and is added to most soft drinks. The primary pharmacological effects of caffeine are as stimulants of the central nervous system, cardiac muscle, and respiratory system. Caffeine also acts as a diuretic (that is, it induces urination). It also delays fatigue. Pharmacologically, it is labeled as a sympathomimetic agent or a pseudostressor. When consumed it triggers a response similar to stress.

Most soft drinks today contain caffeine. According to the National Soft Drink Association, the following is the caffeine content in milligrams per 12-ounce can of soda in some popular products:

Product	*Caffeine Content (mg/12-oz. can)*
Jolt	71.2
Sugar-Free Mr. Pibb	58.8
Mountain Dew	55.0 (no caffeine in Canada)
Diet Mountain Dew	55.0
Kick Citrus	54.0
Mello Yellow	52.8
Surge	51.0
Tab	46.8
Coca-Cola	45.6
Diet Cola	45.6
Shasta Cola	44.4
Shasta Cherry Cola	44.4
Shasta Diet Cola	44.4
Mr. Pibb	40.8
OK Soda	40.5
Dr. Pepper	39.6
Pepsi Cola	37.2
Aspen	36.0
Diet Pepsi	35.4
RC Cola	36.0
Diet RC	36.0
Diet Rite	36.0
Canada Dry Cola	30.0
Canada Dry Diet Cola	1.2
7 Up	0.0

* * * * *

Balanced Diet Plan for Stress Reduction and Healthful Living

The discussion in this chapter has been designed to help you understand the value and importance of maintaining a balanced diet, developing appropriate eating habits, and avoiding negative stress-coping practices like alcohol and drug abuse. Thoughts for Reflection 7.4 will help you to ponder some dietary goals that you need to implement in daily life. Now, sharpen your skills in developing and maintaining a diet plan with the help of Worksheet 7.2.

Thoughts for Reflection 7.4
Dietary Goals to Think About

- To avoid becoming overweight, consume only as much energy (calories) as is expended; if overweight, decrease energy intake and increase energy expenditure.
- Increase the consumption of complex carbohydrates and "naturally occurring" sugars from about 28 percent of energy intake to about 48 percent of energy intake.
- Reduce the consumption of refined and processed sugars by about 45 percent to supply about 10 percent of total energy intake.
- Total fat should be no more than 30 percent of the total calories. Reduce saturated fat consumption to account for no more than 10 percent of total energy intake. Polyunsaturated fats should account for no more than 10 percent of energy intake; monounsaturated fats should make up the remainder (10–15 percent) of total calories.
- Reduce cholesterol consumption to no more than 300 milligrams per day.
- Limit the intake of sodium to 2400 milligrams (2.4 grams per day).

Note: From *Dietary Goals for the United States* (2nd ed.) by Select Committee on Nutrition and Human Needs, 1986, Washington, D.C.: U.S. Senate Select Committee. Material under public domain.

* * * * *

Worksheet 7.2
Ten-Step Balanced Diet Plan for Stress Reduction and Healthful Living

Following are ten steps that will help you plan your diet better for stress reduction and healthful living. Read each step, and in the space provided write your own plan on how you would go about accomplishing that step.

Step 1. **Becoming aware of our dietary habits**

Analyze your dietary habits. Skipping meals intensifies the stress response. The largest meal of the day needs to be taken earlier in the day. Be sure to find out whether you have three meals a day or not. Do you skip any meals? Which is your largest meal of the day?

___

___

___

___

___

___

Step 2. **Establishing a balance among the six food groups**

The U.S. Department of Agriculture's Food Pyramid suggests a balance of six food groups emphasizing bread, grains, vegetables, and fruits, while placing less importance on meat, milk products, fats, and sweets (Figure 7.1). Do you include food items from all six food groups in appropriate quantities?

___

___

___

___

___

___

Worksheet 7.2 Ten-Step Balanced Diet Plan for Stress Reduction and Healthful Living (cont'd)

Step 3. **Planning to limit the intake of caffeinated beverages**

We have already seen that caffeine is a pseudostressor and causes a stresslike response. Therefore, you should work to reduce your intake of caffeinated beverages. Some people like to stop them all at once, whereas others gradually taper their intake, and then substitute their intake with noncaffeinated beverages. Write down and implement a strategy that suits you.

____

____

____

____

____

____

____

Step 4. **Planning to limit the daily intake of salt in your diet**

We have already seen that salt leads to retention of body water and may cause an increase in blood pressure. You need to avoid using any table salt and work at curbing your intake of fast food and precooked food unless it is absolutely necessary. Work out a strategy to implement this plan.

____

____

____

____

____

____

____

Worksheet 7.2 Ten-Step Balanced Diet Plan for Stress Reduction and Healthful Living (cont'd)

Step 5. Planning to limit the daily intake of sugar

Excessive sugar intake can paradoxically reduce the blood levels of sugar, causing hypoglycemia. This result occurs because temporarily high levels of sugar stimulate the release of insulin, which causes blood sugar to fall (Smith, 1993). Therefore, limiting the intake of sugar helps in reducing stress.

____

____

____

____

____

Step 6. Planning to stop smoking

We have seen that smoking does not reduce stress. As discussed earlier, nicotine found in tobacco has an addictive effect on the stress response. To begin with, keeping a record of the number of cigarettes smoked and seeking support from close friends is helpful. You then need to work at delaying the urge to smoke as many times as possible during the day. This purpose can be achieved by diverting the mind to do something else at the time of the urge and replacing the smoking habit with other constructive habits (like exercising). This way you can consistently work at cutting the number of cigarettes you smoke. Finally you need to decide upon a day and quit smoking completely. You need to adhere to this commitment religiously. Work out a definitive plan for yourself to quit smoking.

____

____

____

____

____

____

Worksheet 7.2 Ten-Step Balanced Diet Plan for Stress Reduction and Healthful Living (cont'd)

Step 7. **Planning to avoid or reduce alcohol intake**

Moderation in intake of alcohol and alcoholic beverages is vital in order to maintain balance and avoid stress. If you are not now practicing moderation, begin to work at establishing it.

____

____

____

____

____

____

____

Step 8. **Supplementing vitamins and minerals in the diet**

Establishing a balance in the daily intake of vitamins and minerals in the diet increases resistance to stress. It is best to choose a wide variety of foods to meet one's vitamin and mineral needs in place of supplements (see Table 7.2). Write out a plan to ensure that the needed vitamins and minerals are included in your diet.

____

____

____

____

____

____

____

Worksheet 7.2 Ten-Step Balanced Diet Plan for Stress Reduction and Healthful Living (cont'd)

Step 9. **Utilizing natural food products**

Natural food products like yogurt have been suggested to help improve stress-coping capabilities. One of the components of yogurt, *Lactobacillus acidophilus,* has received attention. These bacteria are harmless and have been claimed to inhibit growth of pathogenic bacteria, boost the immune system, produce essential vitamins, and enhance resistance to stress (Chaitow & Trenev, 1990; Lee, 1988; Schauss, 1990). Plan to increase consumption of natural food products in your diet.

____

____

____

____

____

____

Step 10. **Maintaining weight through regular monitoring and control**

In order to reduce stress in our life, maintaining weight by weekly or bimonthly monitoring and working out an effective diet and exercise plan are vital. What is your plan?

____

____

____

____

____

____

* * * * *

Stress Management Principle 7

Enjoy balanced meals at regular times and cherish the gift.

Summary Points

- Sleeping seven to eight hours daily, eating breakfast daily, consuming only planned snacks between meals, being at or near prescribed height-adjusted weight, never smoking, moderate or no use of alcohol, and regular physical activity are some practices associated with good health.
- A healthy balanced diet when taken at regular times reduces stress and improves upon stress-coping capabilities.
- Maintaining weight based upon the ideal range for height, body frame, and gender is important for healthy living and stress reduction.
- Coffee, tea, and colas have *caffeine,* which is a pseudostressor or a sympathomimetic agent; that is, it produces a stresslike response in the body.
- Nicotine found in tobacco is also a sympathomimetic agent and produces stress.
- Alcohol and illegal drugs do *not* relieve stress but can only add to one's stress.
- Regulating salt and sugar intake in the diet is essential for managing stress.
- USRDA is no more than 2400 milligrams of sodium in the diet per day.
- We need to observe moderation in consuming carbohydrates and proteins in our diet.
- Fats should be used only sparingly.
- Vitamins and minerals should be taken in recommended and optimum quantities.
- Water in the diet is the only constituent that should be taken in unlimited amounts. It is recommended that we drink at least 8–10 glasses of water daily.

References and Further Readings

Belloc, N. B., & Breslow, L. (1972). Relationship of physical health status and health practices. *Preventive Medicine, 1,* 409–421.

Chaitow, L., & Trenev, N. (1990). *Probiotics: The revolutionary "friendly bacteria" way to vital health and well-being.* Northamptonshire: Thorsons.

Cuthbertson, D. P. (1964). Physical injury and its effects on protein metabolism. In H. H. Munro and J. B. Allison (Eds.), *Mammalian protein metabolism,* vol. 2 (pp. 374–414). New York: Academic Press.

Girdano, D. E., Everly, G. S., Jr., Dusek, D. E. (1997). *Controlling stress and tension: A holistic approach* (5th ed.). Englewood Cliffs, NJ: Prentice Hall.

Greenberg, J. S. (1999). *Comprehensive stress management* (6th ed.). Boston: William C. Brown/McGraw-Hill.

Lee, W. H. (1988). *The friendly bacteria: How lactobacilli and bifidobacteria can transform your health.* New Canaan, CT: Keats.

Ray, O., & Ksir, C. (1999). *Drugs, society, and human behavior* (8th ed.). Boston: William C. Brown/McGraw-Hill.

Schauss, A. G. (1990). *Lactobacillus acidophilus:* Method of action, clinical application and toxicity data. *Journal of Advancement in Medicine, 3,* 163–178.

Schlaadt, R. G. (1992). *Alcohol use and abuse.* Guilford, CT: Dushkin.

Seventh Special Report to the U.S. Congress on Alcohol and Health. (1990, January). Department of Health and Human Services, Public Health Service, Alcohol, Drug Abuse, and Mental Health Administration, National Institute on Alcohol Abuse and Alcoholism.

Smith, J. C. (1993). *Understanding stress and coping.* New York: Macmillan.

CHAPTER 8

Regular Exercise and Physical Activity

Better to hunt in fields, for health unbought,
Than fee the doctor for a nauseous draught.
The wise, for cure, on exercise depend;
God never made his work, for man to mend.

—*John Dryden*

Importance of Exercise and Physical Activity

Exercise and physical activity not only are good for physical health but also enhance mental health. Improvement in both these dimensions contributes positively toward coping with stress effectively. Exercise performed regularly promotes health by

- Providing higher energy levels
- Improving bodily resistance to disease
- Improving cardiovascular and respiratory fitness
- Enhancing self-esteem and confidence
- Regulating sleep patterns
- Improving the ability to concentrate
- Increasing strength and stamina
- Bringing about an overall positive and healthy outlook to life

Various studies have supported the usefulness of regular exercise. Paffenberger and colleagues (1993) demonstrated that regular exercise during leisure time can protect people against premature death from any cause, particularly coronary heart disease. The exact mechanism by which exercise operates to reduce the incidence of coronary heart disease is debatable. A number of theories have been presented. Some researchers theorize that it is due to modification of feelings such as anger (Czajkowski et al., 1990); some attribute it to physiological reasons like increased blood flow to the brain or release of endorphins (Smith, 1993); and, finally, others believe it is due to diversion of attention from daily hassles and an accompanying relief in stress (Bahrke & Morgan, 1978). Whatever be the exact mechanism, there is a great deal of positive evidence in support of regular exercise.

In 1996 the U.S. Department of Health and Human Services released the first Surgeon General's Report to address physical activity and health (U.S. Department of Health and Human Services, 1996). The primary message of this report was that Americans can substantially improve their health and quality of life by incorporating moderate amounts of physical activity in their lives. With regard to stress-related disorders, the report pointed out that physical activity appeared to "relieve symptoms of depression and anxiety and improve mood" (pp. 8, 136). In the wake of all these recommendations, it makes a lot of sense to include regular exercise and physical activity in one's lifestyle to reduce stress and manage it better.

Box 8.1 Physical Activity: Benefits and Recommendations from the Surgeon General's Report

Regular physical activity is helpful in preventing and controlling morbidity and premature mortality associated with a number of chronic diseases. The chief benefits of regular physical activity include these:

- Prevention and control of coronary heart disease (CHD), stroke, non-insulin-dependent diabetes mellitus, hypertension (high blood pressure), osteoporosis, colon cancer, depression, anxiety, and obesity
- Improved heart, lung, and circulatory system functioning
- Better balance of blood lipids as a result of increasing "good cholesterol," or high-density lipoproteins (HDL), and lowering "bad cholesterol," or low-density lipoproteins (LDL)
- Improved quality of life
- Enhanced functional independence
- Mental well-being
- Counterbalancing of adverse effects due to stress
- Improved self-esteem
- Maintenance of appropriate body weight
- Slowing down the adverse effects of aging such as memory loss
- Overall improved life expectancy

Current recommendations from the Surgeon General's Report include the following:

- Goal of at least 30 minutes or more of moderate-intensity activities on most days of the week
- Utilization of recreational activities such as jogging, bicycling, and swimming in daily life
- Inclusion of lifestyle activities such as climbing stairs, mowing the lawn, or walking to and from work in everyday routine

* * * * *

Types of Exercise

In order to describe types of exercise, a number of classifications are available. From a *biological* point of view, depending upon the oxygen utilization by the body, exercise can be classified into two types:

1. *Aerobic exercise* (*aerobic* meaning "with oxygen") can be defined as exercise that does not require greater oxygen than can be taken in by the body. Examples of aerobic activities include running, walking briskly, jogging, bicycling, swimming, and rope jumping.

2. *Anaerobic exercise* (*anaerobic* meaning "without oxygen") can be defined as exercise in which the body goes all out and the muscles rely heavily on production of energy without adequate oxygen. Examples of anaerobic activity would be sprinting 100 or 200 meters with maximum effort.

This classification is more theoretical in its connotation. According to a *functional* point of view, exercise can be classified into the following types:

1. *Exercise for Circulatory and Respiratory Fitness.* The circulatory system consists of the heart, blood, and blood vessels. The blood is an important carrier of oxygen to all cells of the body. Oxygen is utilized by the cells to produce necessary energy for daily activities. The respiratory system consists of the airways and lungs. The air that we breathe in is taken up by the lungs, and oxygen is supplied to the blood. Therefore, both the circulatory and the respiratory systems are important in supplying oxygen to provide necessary energy to the body. This plays an important role in managing stress. Examples of activities that improve circulatory and respiratory fitness include brisk walking, jogging, running, and aerobic dancing.

2. *Exercise for Enhancing Muscular Strength and Endurance.* Muscular strength is the ability to achieve maximal performance. Muscular endurance is the ability to work continuously for a long period of time. Examples of activities that improve muscular strength and endurance include push-ups, sit-ups, chin-ups, and weight training.

3. *Exercise for Improving Body Flexibility.* Flexibility is the ability of the body to perform various motions around the joints. Some activities that promote flexibility are stretching, shoulder reach, trunk flexion, trunk extension, and so on.

4. *Exercise for Reducing Body Fat.* Fat is normally deposited around the waist for men and on the thighs for women. Fat deposition also leads to atherosclerotic changes in arteries (narrowing with fatty deposition) and greater risk for coronary heart disease. Generally, exercise activities performed for circulatory and respiratory fitness and muscular strength, described previously, also help in burning off fat.

From an *operational* point of view, which is based upon the method of performance, exercise can be classified as follows:

1. *Interval training* includes exercising in bouts of hard activities separated by bouts of light exercise.

2. *Continuous training* includes exercising at a constant, rhythmic level of intensity for a long and uninterrupted period.

3. *Circuit training* includes completing a round of exercises known as a *circuit.* This "circuit" can be repeated for a desirable length of time and pace.

From an *applied practical* point of view, exercise can be classified as follows:

1. *Competitive* exercise includes performing for the purpose of competition, that is, in order to win an event. This competitive exercise produces great stress for many of us. One way to prevent this type of stress is to avoid competitive sports. If participation in competitive sports is inevitable, or one has a desire to do so, then one has to learn and develop appropriate coping skills in order to avoid potential negative consequences from stress.

2. *Semicompetitive* exercise normally begins as a noncompetitive event, but when one gets into the mood, then one starts competing with others. This competition can also produce stress, and therefore, appropriate skills are required in coping.

3. *Noncompetitive* activities are performed purely for one's own health and satisfaction. There is no element of competition of any kind. This kind of exercise does not produce any negative consequences associated with stress. On the other hand, noncompetitive exercise helps in counteracting the negative consequences of stress.

From the perspective of preventing, reducing, controlling, and managing stress, any noncompetitive, aerobic exercise performed rhythmically, with regularity, is most beneficial. Examples of some activities that meet these criteria are as follows:

- *Jogging and Running.* Jogging and running are quite popular in the United States and very simple to perform. They require no special training and can be performed in almost any location and at any time of the day. All one needs is a good pair of running shoes. One also needs to have an empty stomach, that is, not having eaten anything for at least three to four hours. This activity can be performed individually or in groups. This is an excellent aerobic and rhythmic activity and is excellent for preventing, reducing, and managing stress.

- *Brisk Walking.* For older persons and people not used to exercising, brisk walking can be a very important initiating exercise. A walking technique needs to be natural and rhythmic. Use of correct posture and proper shoes are also important. This is a most inexpensive form of exercise, and if performed regularly, it can yield rich dividends.

- *Cycling.* Cycling is also an aerobic rhythmic, cardiorespiratory exercise and is quite helpful in preventing, reducing, and managing stress. For this purpose cycling needs to be performed noncompetitively either outdoors or in a velodrome. For adequate results this activity needs to be done regularly for 30 minutes, at least three to four times a week.

- *Swimming.* Swimming has often been called the most complete form of exercise. Swimming improves cardiorespiratory fitness, flexibility, muscular strength, and endurance. A significant advantage of swimming is that, since the body is supported by water, risk of harm to joints and muscles is minimal. This activity is an effective means to prevent, reduce, and manage stress.

- *Cross-Country Skiing.* Cross-country skiing also provides cardiorespiratory and muscular benefits. The whole body is utilized when performing this exercise. This activity is also helpful in preventing, reducing, and managing stress. It may appear that this activity can only be performed outdoors in the winter, but this is not so. One can also perform this activity indoors with the help of artificial equipment.

• *Aerobic Dancing.* Aerobic dancing has gained popularity over the past decade. This activity helps the whole body to obtain adequate cardiorespiratory fitness, flexibility, and muscular endurance. In this activity the mind is constantly engaged in achieving rhythmic coordination, and therefore, this focus helps divert attention from stress-producing thoughts.

• *Activities Involving Use of Any Racquet.* Activities such as racquetball, tennis, table tennis, badminton, squash, and so on, if played noncompetitively, are helpful forms of exercise for improving cardiorespiratory fitness, flexibility, muscular strength, and endurance. These activities also relieve one from the potential harmful negative consequences of stress.

Before you proceed to the steps toward initiating and sustaining an exercise program, become more aware of your exercise levels by completing Worksheet 8.1. Worksheet 8.2 will help you to determine target heart rates appropriate for you while performing exercise. Thoughts for Reflection 8.1 will help you become familiar with some principles for conditioning the body.

Worksheet 8.1
Enhancing Self-Awareness about Exercise Levels

Circle the choice that best describes your behavior pertaining to exercise.

	Low		*Moderate*		*High*
1. Level of physical activity at work	1	2	3	4	5
2. Level of physical activity at leisure	1	2	3	4	5
3. Regularity of exercise	1	2	3	4	5
4. Number of times per week	1–2		3–4	5–6	>6
5. Duration of exercise	<15 min.		15–30/30–45 min.		>45 min.

6. Describe the type of exercise you do:

____

____

____

____

____

____

____

____

____

____

____

____

____

____

____

FEEDBACK ON WORKSHEET 8.1

From the point of view of preventing, reducing, controlling and managing stress, exercise needs to be rhythmic, aerobic, noncompetitive, and performed for an adequate amount of time. This worksheet should have provided you with insight on your behavior pertaining to exercise. If your exercise levels are low, then you need to increase them. If your exercise levels are already high, then you need to sustain these efforts and attain regularity.

If the types of exercise you are performing are not holistic, that is, if they do not contribute much to all the dimensions including cardiorespiratory fitness, flexibility, muscular strength, and endurance, then you need to choose activities that contribute to all the dimensions. Some activities that have been described earlier include jogging/running, brisk walking, cycling, swimming, cross-country skiing, aerobic dancing, and activities involving the use of a racquet. You should remember to include the components of rhythm, aerobics, and regularity in your exercise schedule.

* * * * *

Worksheet 8.2
Calculating Appropriate Target Heart-Rate Range

In order for an exercise to produce optimum benefits for cardiorespiratory fitness and prevention of stress, exercise levels need to reach target heart rate for at least 15–30 minutes. In order to calculate your target heart-rate range for exercising, proceed as follows:

1. Subtract your age from 220. Call this *A*.

   220 – Your age = _______ (*A*)

2. Take your pulse in a resting state for one minute. It is best to record one's pulse before getting up from bed in the morning to get a true resting heart rate. You can feel the radial pulse at the wrist toward the side of the thumb (against the neck of the radius bone) or the carotid pulse in the neck against the Adam's apple. Use your ring finger to feel the pulse so that there is no confusion with the pulse in the thumb, index, or middle fingers. Call this *B*, and write it down in the following space.

   B = _______ beats per minute

3. Subtract *B* from *A*. Call this *C*.

   A – *B* = _______ – _______ = _______ (C)

4. Multiply C by 0.6. Call the result *D*.

   C × 0.6 = _______ × 0.6 = _______ (*D*)

5. Add *B* and *D* to obtain the *lower end* of your target heart rate range.

   B + *D* = _______ + _______ = _______

6. Multiply C by 0.8. Call the result *E*.

   C × 0.8 = _______ × 0.8 = _______ (*E*)

7. Add *B* and *E* to obtain the *upper end* of your target heart rate range.

   B + *E* = _______ + _______ = _______

FEEDBACK ON WORKSHEET 8.2

This worksheet should have provided you with an appropriate target heart rate range specific for your age. While exercising, it is extremely important to adhere to this target heart range and not exceed the upper limit at any time. This target heart range can be monitored while performing the exercise by taking your own pulse. If you are exceeding the target heart range, then you need to slow down. Another "rough" method of estimating this is the "talk test." According to this test, if you are able to maintain normal conversation while exercising, then you are within the target heart range.

You need to remain within the target heart range for 15–30 minutes in the conditioning phase of the exercise. Only after regular exercise for over six months to one year can this period be exceeded. We recommend that you do not exceed this period unless you want to become a professional athlete.

It is also important to slowly and *not* suddenly achieve the target heart range. That is why it is recommended that you initiate any exercise activity with *warming up and stretching.* It is equally important to slowly and not suddenly turn back to the normal heart range after being in the target heart range for 15–30 minutes. Therefore, it is recommended that you end any exercise activity with a slow *cooldown.* This caution acquires greater significance as you grow older.

* * * * *

Thoughts for Reflection 8.1
Principles of Conditioning for Exercise

Conditioning the Mind

- Think about the benefits of an exercise program.
- Try to visualize what an exercise program can do for you.
- You have to find time to exercise. You can find sufficient time for exercise even if your schedule is extremely busy. Time availability needs to be created in the mind first.
- Think of any friends or family members who can help you to monitor your exercise. Enter into an agreement with them.
- Be prepared to face a little discomfort in the form of aches and pains in the beginning when you initiate an exercise program.

Conditioning the Body

- Increase your exercise levels *slowly*. You should not initiate vigorous exercise suddenly. It's best to build up exercise levels slowly and gradually.
- You should remember to start an exercise program with *warming up* your body for at least 10 minutes. This includes activities performed at a slower pace.
- After the warming-up phase you can go into the *conditioning* phase. You have to be careful not to overdo this phase. One of the criteria for judging the intensity is to find your *target heart rate* (see Worksheet 8.2) and not exceed this rate for 15–30 minutes.
- You always have to remember to *cool down* for 5–10 minutes after the intensive conditioning phase so that the heart rate comes back to near normal. Any easy-paced activity will help you to cool down after the strenuous conditioning phase.
- Maintaining regularity in exercising is vital for achieving maximum benefits.

* * * * *

Initiating and Sustaining an Exercise Program

We have discussed the importance and types of exercise, and we have enhanced our awareness regarding our exercise levels. We have also familiarized ourselves with the various principles required for conditioning the body and mind in order to prepare for exercise. Now we need to work toward initiating and sustaining regular exercise activities. Worksheet 8.3 has been designed to facilitate achieving this regularity. It is hoped that this worksheet will foster insights into your behavior and help you adopt an exercise lifestyle. Thoughts for Reflection 8.2 presents some cautions that you need to keep in mind before, during, and after exercise.

Worksheet 8.3
Five Steps toward Initiation and Sustenance of an Exercise Program

Following are five steps that will help you initiate and sustain an exercise program. Read the text associated with each step. In the space provided, write down your own plan as to how you would go about accomplishing that step.

Step 1. **Determining your exercise levels**

An awareness about your exercise levels is the first step toward developing your own plan of improvement. In the space provided, based upon feedback from Worksheet 8.1, rate your exercise levels and write down what, how, and how much you need to improve.

____

____

____

____

Step 2. **Checking before exercise**

Before proceeding to initiate an exercise program, respond to the following questions. If you answer yes or are not sure about any of the following questions, you should consult your physician before beginning an exercise program.

- Is there a history of any heart disease in my family?

  _______ Yes _______ No _______ Not sure

- Have I ever been diagnosed to have any heart disease?

  _______ Yes _______ No _______ Not sure

- Have I ever suffered from chest pains?

  _______ Yes _______ No _______ Not sure

- Do I have shortness of breath while climbing up a flight of stairs?

  _______ Yes _______ No _______ Not sure

Worksheet 8.3 Five Steps toward Initiation and Sustenance of an Exercise Program (cont'd)

- Have I ever been diagnosed to have diabetes mellitus, or had high blood sugar or sugar in urine detected, or had complaints of excessive hunger, thirst, or increased urination?

  ________ Yes ________ No ________ Not sure

- Am I a smoker?

  ________ Yes ________ No ________ Not sure

- Am I over 35 years of age and have not exercised regularly?

  ________ Yes ________ No ________ Not sure

- Have I ever been diagnosed to have high serum cholesterol levels (particularly LDL or "bad cholesterol")?

  ________ Yes ________ No ________ Not sure

- Am I taking any prescribed medication(s)?

  ________ Yes ________ No ________ Not sure

- Do I have any other medical problems or disabilities?

  ________ Yes ________ No ________ Not sure

***Step* 3. Starting an exercise program**

Having decided that you want to initiate an exercise program, you have to choose an appropriate place. Exercise either early in the morning when your stomach is empty or late in the afternoon before dinner. It is important to remember that exercise habits need to be changed gradually. You should increase duration by one to five minutes every other session.

Worksheet 8.3 Five Steps toward Initiation and Sustenance of an Exercise Program (cont'd)

An exercise program always has three parts: *warm-up, conditioning,* and *cooldown.* You should practice all three stages meticulously. Now is the time to make a plan to start your exercise program if you do not already have one.

____

____

____

____

____

____

____

Step 4. **Braving the initial "teething" problems**

It is usual to have pain, discomfort, and tiredness in the initial few days of starting an exercise plan. To be prepared for these, write down in the following space all the anticipated problems you are likely to face and how you are going to manage them. This step will help you adapt to change in your exercise plan.

____

____

____

____

____

____

____

____

Worksheet 8.3 Five Steps toward Initiation and Sustenance of an Exercise Program (cont'd)

***Step 5.* Sustaining regularity in exercise**

Just as the plant in the pot withers away without regular replenishment by water, any good habit, if not incorporated into a regular plan, does not provide us with complete benefits. Now you should make a plan for yourself as to how you would like to sustain your exercise program.

____

____

____

____

____

____

____

____

____

* * * * *

Thoughts for Reflection 8.2
Cautions with Exercise

- You should not start vigorous exercise suddenly. You have to make a plan before you implement it.
- You have to be careful not to overexert. Common signs of overexertion are

  Frequent headaches.

  Breathing difficulties and shortness of breath.

  Excessive tiredness and fatigue that last a long time.

  Nausea or vomiting after exercise.

  Severe pain all over the body, especially in overworked muscles.

  Inability to perform daily activities.

  Excessive strain of any part of the body.
- Be aware of abnormal signs when exercising. Common abnormal signs are

  Chest pain.

  Dizziness, fainting.

  Fits.

  Irregular heart movements as felt by palpitations.

  Sustained pain in the joints.

  Swelling in any part of the body after exercise.
- Drink plenty of water and fluids with electrolytes to avoid getting dehydrated.
- Do not exercise when your stomach is full. You should wait at least 2 hours before exercising if you have eaten something.
- During pregnancy, the expectant mother should consult her physician before following a regular exercise schedule.
- Wear a comfortable outfit. Do not wear very tight clothes. Your shoes need to be selected carefully and not cause blisters, corns, or sores.

* * * * *

Stress Management Principle 8

Start an exercise program and keep exercising regularly.

Summary Points

- Regular exercise promotes health by providing higher energy levels, improving body resistance to disease, enhancing self-esteem and confidence, increasing strength and stamina, and bringing about an overall positive and healthy outlook to life.
- Regular exercise helps to prevent, reduce, control, and manage stress.
- Biologically, exercise can be classified as aerobic and anaerobic.
- Functionally, exercise can be classified as activities improving cardiorespiratory fitness, activities enhancing muscular strength and endurance, activities improving body flexibility, and activities reducing fat.
- Operationally, exercise can be classified as interval, continuous, and circuit training.
- Practically, exercise can be classified as competitive, semicompetitive, and noncompetitive.
- In order for exercise to produce optimum benefits for cardiorespiratory fitness and for prevention, reduction, and management of stress, the exercise levels need to reach target heart rate for at least 15–30 minutes.
- Conditioning the body and mind are prerequisites for initiating and sustaining any exercise program.
- Steps of an ideal exercise program include *warm-up* (10 minutes), *conditioning* (maintaining the target heart rate for 15–30 minutes), and *cooldown* (10 minutes).
- Regularity in exercising is extremely important in order to obtain maximum benefits.

References and Further Readings

Bahrke, M. S., & Morgan, W. P. (1978). Anxiety reduction following exercise and meditation. *Cognitive Therapy and Research, 2,* 323–333.

Czajkowski, S. M., Hindelang, R. D., Dembroski, T. M., Mayerson, S. E., Parks, E. B., & Holland, J. C. (1990). Aerobic fitness, psychological characteristics, and cardiovascular reactivity to stress. *Health psychology, 9,* 676–692.

Girdano, D. E., Everly, G. S., Jr., & Dusek, D. E. (1997). *Controlling stress and tension: A holistic approach* (5th ed.). Englewood Cliffs, NJ: Prentice Hall.

Greenberg, J. S. (1999). *Comprehensive stress management* (6th ed.). Boston: William C. Brown/McGraw-Hill.

Paffenberger, R. S., Jr., Hyde, R. T., Wing, A. L., Lee, I. M., Jung, D. L., & Kampert, J. B. (1993). The association of changes in physical activity level and other lifestyle characteristics with mortality among men. *New England Journal of Medicine, 328,* 538–545.

Smith, J. C. (1993). *Understanding stress and coping.* New York: Macmillan.

U.S. Department of Health and Human Services. (1996). *Physical activity and health: A Report of the Surgeon General.* Atlanta, GA: USDHHS, Centers for Disease Control and Prevention, National Center for Chronic Disease Prevention and Health Promotion.

CHAPTER 9

Efficient Time Management

To Daffodils

Fair daffodils, we weep to see
You haste away so soon:
As yet the early-rising sun
Has not attain'd his noon.
Stay, stay,
Until the hasting day
Has run
But to the evensong;
And, having pray'd together, we
Will go with you along.
We have short time to stay, as you,
We have as short a spring;
As quick a growth to meet decay,
As you or anything.

—Robert Herrick

Importance of Time Management

Time is one of our most precious resources. All of us have the same time available to us, and this time is limited. Our existence on Earth has a limited time frame. We are not even aware how much time is available in our life. Therefore, we need to make the best use of whatever time is available to us. Moreover, the way we utilize this time determines success in accomplishing our desired goals. In present times this success is an important determinant of our happiness and peace of mind. If we utilize our time judiciously and efficiently, we can become more successful. However, if we are unable to utilize our time appropriately, our productivity is decreased. This inefficiency in managing our time may create problems. It leads to unfulfillment of our expectations and desired goals, which in turn can become a great source of stress for us. Therefore, management of time efficiently and effectively acquires great significance.

Another important dimension with regard to utilization of our time is to have appropriate *balance* in our activities. We need to allocate adequate time for physical activities, mental enrichment, social interactions, and spiritual well-being. All these dimensions are important spokes of a "holistic wheel" for harmony in life as shown in Figure 9.1.

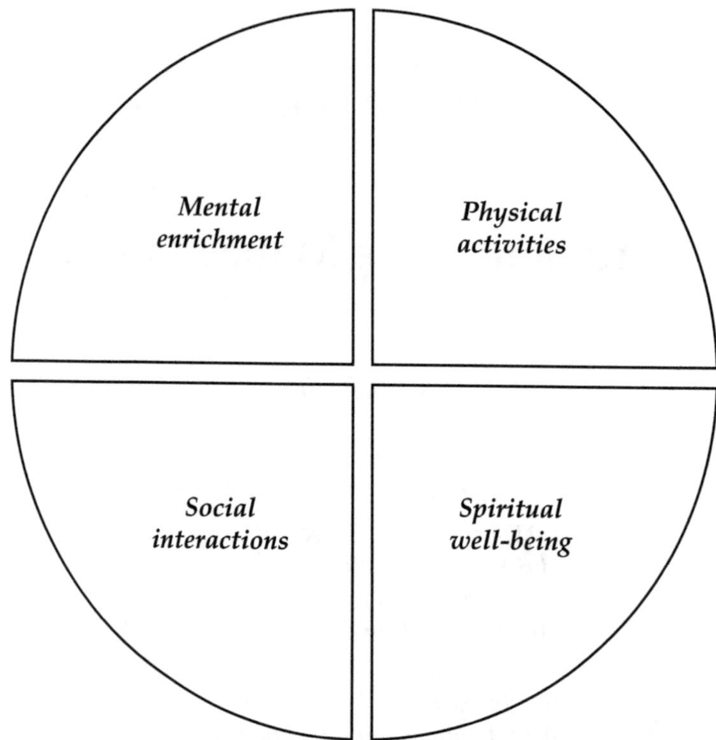

Figure 9.1 "Holistic Wheel" of Harmony in Life

One popular management principle, in the context of time management, is the *Pareto principle.* According to this principle, most of the desired key results are obtained by only a few of our total activities. On the other hand, the majority of other activities generate only a few of the key results. Pareto estimated that this relationship was 20 percent to 80 percent in most situations; that is, 80 percent of the results would be derived from 20 percent of the objectives, while 80 percent of the objectives would yield only 20 percent of the results. Therefore, *priority* of effort may be given to those objectives identified as *the critical few* (Liebler, Levine, & Rothman, 1992). This approach of learning and practicing to prioritize our daily activities and tasks, in order to optimize results, will be the basis for our discussion on efficient time management.

Manifestations of Poor Time Management

Poor time management seems to be a "universal" problem. It is generally shown from studies on time management that the majority of us, most of the time, admit to not managing our time very well and acknowledge that this failure creates stress in our lives. Some of the manifestations of poor time management are as follows:

- Unfulfilled expectations
- Inability to be on time for appointments

- Hurrying to be on time
- Poor planning
- Inability to achieve desired objectives
- Tiredness and fatigue resulting from unplanned downtime
- Regret over missed deadlines
- Disappointments
- Inadequate time for rest
- Borrowing time from time slots for family, work, leisure, free time, or personal relationships
- Constant feeling of being overwhelmed
- Feeling of "too much going on"
- Worrying about how to get things done
- Inability to deliver goods on time
- Insecure feelings about the future
- Regrets about the past

Therefore, poor time management is an important source of stress and leads to negative harmful consequences. These undue negative consequences are self-inflicted and can be easily prevented if we understand, apply, and follow the basic principles of time management.

Self-understanding is a prerequisite to making any change, particularly in changing our behavior in relation to efficient time management (Januz & Jones, 1981). Therefore, before you proceed to learn about the basic principles of efficient time management, you need to gain an insight into your own behavior and find out whether managing time is a problem for you. This understanding will provide you with a benchmark as to where you can start your efforts at managing time efficiently and effectively. Worksheet 9.1 has been designed to help you enhance this understanding. Thoughts for Reflection 9.1 will help you to ponder some of the barriers that may be preventing you from managing your time efficiently.

Box 9.1 Time Waster Personalities

Professor Brian Seaward (1994) in his book on managing stress describes six personalities that can be classified as time wasters:

1. *Type A Personalities.* The characteristics of the Type A personality are described in Chapter 1. On the surface, Type A personality people may appear to be organized and productive, but evidence points to the contrary. These people, in their pursuit for competition, tend to complete tasks in a hurry, spend time in hostility, and try to perform several tasks at one time, all of which amount to time wastage.

2. *Workaholics.* Workaholics tend to derive satisfaction from long work hours. In essence, these people tend to do trivial tasks in normal work hours and major projects after hours, do not use time saving measures, and derive pleasure in working long hours, all of which amount to time wastage.

3. *Time Jugglers.* Time jugglers try to perform more than one thing at a time. Have you ever seen a person who is driving, using a cell phone, grabbing a sandwich, and soothing a child in the rear seat—all at the same time? These people tend to begin several tasks without reaching closure on any, miss out on important responsibilities, and spend more time than needed on tasks—thus making them time wasters.

4. *Procrastinators.* Procrastinators apply diversion tactics and put off what needs to be done today. They tend to do *less difficult* tasks rather than *important* tasks, take a stab at the task but find an excuse to drift away from completing it, and knowingly do things other than the job at hand, all of which amount to wastage of time.

5. *Perfectionists.* Perfectionists are obsessed with carrying out every task to perfection. They get caught in detail, never see the big picture, are too hard on themselves and others, and perform the same task repeatedly, all of which add to time wastage.

6. *Lifestyle Behavior Trappers.* Lifestyle behavior trappers have a hard time saying no. Since they have other people's agendas thrust upon them, they never make efforts at organizing their tasks. They look for gratification from others and they end up wasting time.

* * * * *

Worksheet 9.1
Enhancing Awareness of How You Spend Your Time

Sit down, relax, and respond to the following questions honestly. There are no right or wrong answers. This worksheet will enhance your awareness about how you are using your time.

1. In the past week, was I late for any appointment(s)?

   ____ Yes ____ No ____ Not sure

   If yes, how many times? ____ out of ____ times.

   Reasons:

   ____

   ____

   ____

2. In the past week, did I miss my breakfast, lunch, or supper in order to be on time for some task?

   ____ Yes ____ No ____ Not sure

   If yes, how many times? ____ out of 21 times.

   Reasons:

   ____

   ____

   ____

3. Do I feel lethargic or tired often?

   ____ Yes ____ No ____ Not sure

   If yes, what do you think causes this feeling?

   ____

   ____

   ____

Worksheet 9.1 Enhancing Awareness of How You Spend Your Time (cont'd)

4. In the past week, did I miss any deadline at work or any other personal obligation?

 ____ Yes ____ No ____ Not sure

 If yes, when?

 ____

 Reasons:

 ____

 ____

 ____

5. Am I content with the amount of time that I am devoting to rest and sleep?

 ____ Yes ____ No ____ Not sure

 Reasons:

 ____

 ____

 ____

6. In the past week, did I ever feel that "too much was going on" in my life?

 ____ Yes ____ No ____ Not sure

 If yes, when?

 ____

 Reasons:

 ____

 ____

 ____

Worksheet 9.1 Enhancing Awareness of How You Spend Your Time (cont'd)

7. How much time do I give for:

	Too Much	*Enough*	*Not Adequate*
Work			
Family			
Personal relationships/ friends			
Exercise			
My own free time			
Leisure and recreation			

8. Do I consider myself being overwhelmed at the present moment in my life?

____ Yes ____ No ____ Not sure

Reasons:

____

____

____

____

____

____

____

____

____

Worksheet 9.1 Enhancing Awareness of How You Spend Your Time (cont'd)

9. In the past week, was I able to accomplish all my duties satisfactorily and in a timely manner?

    ____ Yes ____ No ____ Not sure

    Reasons:

    ____

    ____

    ____

10. Do I manage my time well?

    ____ Yes ____ No ____ Not sure

    Reasons:

    ____

    ____

    ____

FEEDBACK ON WORKSHEET 9.1

Now that you have completed Worksheet 9.1 you have acquired an awareness of how you are spending your time. If time management appears to be a problem for you, you will have to strive hard to manage your time more efficiently. This chapter will provide you with some ideas for managing your time more efficiently. These ideas can only serve as possible guidelines. The ultimate decision and actions to be taken have to come from within you. Only you can make a difference as to how efficiently you will manage your time.

* * * * *

Thoughts for Reflection 9.1
Barriers to Efficient Time Management

- *Inability to Prioritize.* If we are not familiar with the basic principles of prioritization, or do not have the necessary skills, or are not willing to prioritize, then any of these situations will act as a barrier to efficient time management. Prioritizing daily activities, short-term objectives, and long-term goals is central to efficient time management.

- *Inability to Say No.* It is simply not possible to please everyone. Nor is it possible to please some people all the time. Therefore, the ability to say no to others if we want to say no, even if it may be somewhat displeasing, is an important practice in efficiently managing our time. This allows us to accomplish our goals and objectives and not become distracted.

- *Imbalance in Life.* We may be neglecting or overindulging in some of our daily activities. We may be overactive physically while neglecting our mental enrichment. Or we may be socially very active but have low levels of physical activity. Or we may be completely "bankrupt" spiritually. Or we may be involved in too many mental activities, so that we become isolated socially. We need balance in life.

- *Too Many Improperly Planned Desires.* The mind is a very powerful source of generating desires. There is nothing wrong with having desires per se, but if we do not have a proper plan to accomplish these desires, then they do more harm than good. We need to select a few key desires, make a plan to achieve them, and work at the plan.

- *Lack of Focus.* If we are not focused on our goals, we will most often spend our time on misdirected activities. We need to think and decide what we want to achieve and then make focused efforts in order to optimize the use of our time.

- *Procrastination.* The habit of delaying accomplishments of any task to the very last minute is an important barrier in efficient time management. Once we know what we need to do, we need to accomplish it as soon as possible.

* * * * *

Approaches to Time Management

Time management has acquired greater significance in modern times. Never before in history has time management been given such importance. Present life has become much more fast paced than in the past. Therefore, approaches for time management need to address present times. A plethora of ideas have been suggested for time management (Assagioli, 1973; Davis, Eshelman, & McKay, 1988; Eliot & Breo, 1989; Greenberg, 1999; Greenwald, 1973; Lakein, 1973; Levinson, 1990; Mackenzie, 1972; Smith, 1993; Swindoll, 1982). In essence, all these approaches to time management emphasize the need to *prioritize* our daily activities and implement a plan to achieve them. From a practical point of view, the basic technique consists of the following components:

- Developing awareness about how one spends one's time
- Setting long-term goals
- Identifying short-term objectives to accomplish these goals
- Establishing priorities
- Concrete decision making about key priorities
- Realistic scheduling and elimination of low priorities
- Overcoming possible barriers
- Implementing the plan of priorities to manage time efficiently

This basic technique of time management helps us in achieving our long-term goals, as well as assists us in accomplishing our daily activities. Developing a longer time horizon is important from a future perspective, while accomplishment of daily activities is important from a present perspective. Both these dimensions play an important role in preventing and reducing undue stress in our life. In this chapter we shall be focusing primarily on managing time with respect to accomplishing daily activities and tasks. The skills pertaining to setting goals and objectives are elaborated on in Chapter 10. Therefore, in this chapter we shall not discuss what goals to set and how to define objectives in meeting those goals. We will assume that goals have already been set, and from there we will elaborate on a practical technique for managing time for accomplishing daily activities and tasks. You may now complete Worksheet 9.2, which has been designed for this purpose. You also need to ponder Thoughts for Reflection 9.2, which will help you appreciate the importance of having time for yourself and focusing on the present. Thoughts for Reflection 9.3 provides some ideas on how you can save time.

Thoughts for Reflection 9.2
It Has Been Quite Some Time . . .

It has been quite some time since I have noticed nature and its beauty around me. When was the last time I looked upon and pondered the blue, beautiful, magnanimous sky, the majestic snow-peaked tall mountains, the green thick forests, the bright shining sun, or other beauties of nature.

It has been even longer since I reflected on the daily intricate and seemingly small events around me. When was the last time I noticed a child's smile, a gesture of kindness by people around me, a token of appreciation, or other gifts of human love.

Rather, I have been too busy with daily hassles—meeting deadlines, fulfilling obligations, yielding to demands, and chasing desires. I have been either regretting past events or worrying about future happenings.

- Am I doing the right thing?
- Am I utilizing my time wisely?
- Am I happy, contented, and satisfied?
- Do I have peace of mind?

Two issues seem apparent. First, I have not taken enough time for myself. Second, I have ignored the most important frontier, "the now!" I have not completely understood the true value of "today" and the importance of having time available for myself. I need to reflect and restore the inherent joy of having *time for myself now.*

* * * * *

Worksheet 9.2
Practical Steps to Time Management

Seek out a quiet place and complete the following worksheet. You can photocopy this worksheet if you require more space.

***Step 1.* Developing awareness about how you are currently spending your time**

Worksheet 9.1 has already provided you with some insights. Now you can summarize those findings in a chronological and meaningful sequence in the space provided here:

Past one week:

Activities desired	Activities performed

Past one month:

Activities desired	Activities performed

Worksheet 9.2 Practical Steps to Time Management (cont'd)

Past one year:

Activities desired	Activities performed

A comparison between the activities desired and performed will provide you with an understanding of the gap that exists and needs to be rectified.

***Step* 2. List of all desired activities**

Now, make a comprehensive list of all the activities that you need to accomplish in a chronological manner.

Today:

____

____

____

____

____

____

____

____

____

Worksheet 9.2 Practical Steps to Time Management (cont'd)

Within the next week:

Within the next month:

Within the next year:

Worksheet 9.2 Practical Steps to Time Management (cont'd)

***Step 3.* Establishing priorities**

Now you should ask yourself, "What is the best use of my time right now?" Having reflected upon this question, you need to classify all desired activities into three categories: A, high value (activities that need to be done absolutely and immediately), B, medium value (activities that need to be accomplished as soon as possible), and C, low value (activities that need to be done at some time or may even be ignored).

	Category A	*Category B*	*Category C*
Today:			
Within the next week:			
Within the next month:			
Within the next year:			

Worksheet 9.2 Practical Steps to Time Management (cont'd)

Step 4. **Reassessing priorities**

Every day before going to bed, you need to reassess the priorities set in Step 3 and see which ones remain unfulfilled. You should identify any obstacles or barriers that may have been responsible. Then you need to make necessary changes. You can record your observations in the space provided:

____

____

____

____

____

____

____

FEEDBACK ON WORKSHEET 9.2

This worksheet should have helped you prioritize your daily activities as well as possible activities in the near future. You need to make focused efforts at achieving activities listed in Category A. After having accomplished the activities in Category A, you need to proceed to complete the activities listed in Category B. Only after accomplishing tasks in these activities should you look at tasks in Category C, even though they may appear to be simple and easy. You should not be allured by this simplicity, and you should focus only on the importance of the activities.

* * * * *

Thoughts for Reflection 9.3
Ways You Can Save Time

- Establish priorities.
- Adhere to established priorities.
- Avoid procrastination.
- Avoid gossip.
- Have a balance in types of activities.
- Avoid unnecessary socialization.
- Self-organize.
- Delegate tasks.
- Do not always seek perfection.
- Have faith in the ability of others.
- Overcome undue frustration.
- Simplify the tasks.
- Refuse when you would like to refuse.
- Have free time to reflect and plan.
- Think before doing.
- Do not overindulge in only pleasure-seeking activities.
- Make written lists of daily tasks to be done.

* * * * *

STRESS MANAGEMENT PRINCIPLE 9

Do it now!

Summary Points

- Time is a precious resource that needs to be managed efficiently and effectively.
- We need to have appropriate balance in our physical activities, mental enrichment, social interactions, and spiritual well-being.
- According to Pareto's principle, most of our desired key results are obtained by only a few of our activities, while the majority of our activities generate only a few key results. Usually this ratio is 80:20.
- Some manifestations of poor time management include unfulfilled expectations, inability to be on time for appointments, hurrying, disappointment, regrets, and so on.
- Self-understanding is a prerequisite to efficient time management.
- Barriers to efficient time management include inability to prioritize, inability to say no, imbalance in life, too many improperly planned desires, lack of focus, and procrastination.
- Central to all approaches to time management is the understanding and practice of the skill to prioritize.
- There are two important things for peace and happiness: having time for oneself and focusing on the present.

References and Further Readings

Assagioli, R. (1973). *The act of will.* New York: Viking Press.

Burke, C. R., Hall, D. R., & Hawley, D. (1986). *Living with stress.* Clackamas, OR: Wellsource.

Davis, M., Eshelman, E. R., & McKay, M. (1988). *The relaxation and stress reduction workbook* (3rd ed.). Oakland, CA: New Harbinger.

Eliot, R. S., & Breo, D. L. (1989). *Is it worth dying for? How to make stress work for you—not against you* (rev. ed.) (p. 216). New York: Bantam.

Greenberg, J. S. (1999). *Comprehensive stress management* (6th ed.). Boston: William C. Brown/McGraw-Hill.

Greenwald, H. (1973). *Direct decision therapy.* San Diego: EDITS.

Hanson, P. G. (1986). *The joy of stress.* New York: Andrews and McNeal.

Januz, L. R., & Jones, S. K. (1981). *Time management for executives.* New York: Scribner's.

Lakein, A. (1973). *How to get control of your time and your life.* New York: Signet.

Levinson, J. C. (1990). *The ninety-minute hour.* New York: E. P. Dutton.

Liebler, J. G., Levine, R. E., & Rothman, J. (1992). *Management principles for health professionals* (2nd ed.). Gaithersburg, MD: Aspen.

Mackenzie, A. (1972). *The time trap.* New York: AMACOM.

Rice, P. L. (1999). *Stress and health* (3rd ed.). Belmont, CA: Wadsworth.

Seaward, B. L. (1994). *Managing stress: Principles and strategies for health and well being.* Boston: Jones and Bartlett.

Smith, J. C. (1993). *Creative stress management: The 1-2-3 cope system.* Englewood Cliffs, NJ: Prentice Hall.

Swindoll, C. R. (1982). *Strengthening your grip: How to live confidently in an aimless world.* Dallas: Word.

CHAPTER 10

Implementing a Stress Reduction Plan

Rabbi Ben Ezra

Grow old along with me!
The best is yet to be,
The last of life, for which the first was made:
Our times are in His hand
Who saith, "A whole I planned,
Youth shows but half; trust God: see all, nor be afraid!"

—*Robert Browning*

Importance of Implementing a Plan

Any intention—however noble it may be, any plan—however well conceived it may be, any desire—however chaste it may be, *unless implemented,* cannot produce the necessary results. We need to implement our intentions, plans, and desires in order to obtain the necessary results. The purpose of this workbook has been to provide us with practical suggestions toward preventing, reducing, and managing the harmful and negative consequences of stress in our daily lives and enabling us to effectively manage changes that are an inevitable part of our life. These practical suggestions, if not implemented in our lives, will be meaningless. We need to make conscious efforts at integrating these suggestions in our daily activities. These efforts will foster positive health and promote our well-being.

The starting point in the process of implementation is to take stock of the resources that are available to us. In implementing a stress reduction plan, a prerequisite is to have *self-motivation.* Unless and until we are motivated to bring about change in our lives, nobody can force us to make that change. We need to be committed. We need to have faith in ourselves and the techniques that we are going to implement. We also need to be aware of what needs to be changed.

Another prerequisite for success is the *degree of changeability* in what it is that we intend to change in our behavior. This changeability varies from individual to individual and is person specific. For example, applying relaxation techniques may be more changeable for some of us while difficult for others who have a more rigid lifestyle, or applying anxiety-coping techniques may be more changeable for some of us while others may find it more difficult, and so on. From a practical point of view, we need to prioritize and put our efforts into those behavior patterns that are *changeable* and *important* (Green & Kreuter, 1991). We need to identify for ourselves, on our own, which behaviors are less changeable and which behaviors are more changeable for us, and which behaviors are more important and which behaviors are less important for us. The behaviors that are more important and more changeable need our first priority. Then we need to alter behaviors that are more important but less changeable. After accomplishing these two sets of behaviors, we can tackle behaviors that are less important and more changeable. Behaviors that are less important and less changeable need to be ignored. This aspect will be presented in Worksheet 10.2 later on in the chapter.

After having this requisite motivation and conditioning, we need to identify the friends, coworkers, family members, associates, and so on who help us in our efforts to implement our stress reduction plan. We need to take them into confidence and share our plan. We need to solicit their support in helping us adhere to the plan. They will provide us with necessary mental, emotional, and social support that will help to keep us from deviating from our decisions. We also need to procure any special accessories or equipment required for implementing the desired set of behaviors. For example, for a cross-country skiing program, we need to have ski gear, appropriate clothing, conditioning, and location.

We also need to make definitive time allocations for implementing our plan. This requirement will entail scheduling the activities for desired behaviors (as suggested in several worksheets throughout this workbook) into our daily plan however busy we may apparently be. We need to allocate regular "blocks of time" for implementing techniques for prevention, reduction, and management of stress.

Finally, we need to make this stress reduction plan fit into our overall scheme of life. To do so, we need to have clarity about where we want to be, or in other words—what is our goal? We also need to have clarity as to how we will achieve this goal, that is, which objectives will lead us to that goal.

Determining Goals, Objectives, and Targets

Goal Setting

Goals are the sum total of projections of our long-term plans. Goals are an indication of what we want to accomplish in our lives. Goals signify a mission, an ambition, a purpose, and overall aim in life. These goals are oftentimes broad in nature. We need to identify goals for ourselves in different spheres of life, namely *personal, professional, social,* and *spiritual.* An example of a personal goal would be achieving personal happiness and peace of mind; an example of a professional goal could be achieving a certain position within an organization; an example of a social goal could be marital contentment; and an example of a spiritual goal could be achieving world peace. Attaining goals within all these spheres is important from the perspective of deriving balance, harmony, and satisfaction in life. If any of these components is missing, then life will not be holistic and complete happiness will elude us. A person without goals is also likely to have greater stress in life because of undirected, aimless efforts.

"Goal analysis" or "goal setting" is a procedure useful in helping us describe the meaning of what we want to achieve in terms of attitude and understanding (Mager, 1972). The concept of setting goals implies that it is not necessarily important to achieve things in the "right way" but to do the "right things." An understanding of what these "right things" are for us is central to goal setting. The sense of direction in our activities is essentially an internally driven behavior. A number of theories have been presented to explain this behavior. One of the most popular theories in psychology, Maslow's *hierarchy of needs theory* on motivation (Maslow, 1954, 1962), identifies the following five levels of needs:

1. Physiological (food, clothing, shelter, sex, and so on)
2. Security and safety (protection from physical and emotional harm)
3. Love, affection, belonging, and social acceptance
4. Self-esteem (internal factors like self-respect, autonomy, and achievement and external factors such as status, recognition, attention, and so on)
5. Self-actualization (to achieve one's maximum potential)

According to Maslow a person progresses from lower level needs, such as physiological and security and safety, to higher level needs, such as self-esteem and self-actualization, during the course of one's lifetime. He hypothesized that the ultimate goal in life for all human beings was to reach self-actualization. According to this theory, it was important to accomplish a lower level of need before proceeding to the next level.

However, later research led to a modification of this theory. Clayton Alderfer (1969) revised this concept and presented an *ERG theory*. ERG is an acronym of the words *existence, relatedness,* and *growth.* These are the three groups of core needs. *Existence* is concerned with basic material requirements (same as Maslow's physiological and safety needs); *relatedness* is similar to Maslow's love need and the external component of Maslow's self-esteem classification; and *growth* is similar to the internal self-esteem component and self-actualization of Maslow's theory. However, the key features that differentiate this ERG theory from Maslow's theory are as follows: (1) more than one level of need may be operative at the same time, and (2) if gratification of a higher level need is blocked, then the desire to satisfy a lower level need is increased. This ERG theory has greater scientific validation (Robbins, 1998).

This basic understanding of motivation is important in enabling us to set our goals. We need to be conscious about the "level of need" operating within our mind at any time. We also need to understand that the ultimate goal in life is to achieve our maximum potential or self-actualization.

Establishing Objectives

Objectives can be defined as concerted, directed, focused step-by-step efforts to achieve goals. Objectives are more precise than goals and represent smaller steps. Some of the attributes in establishing objectives are as follows:

- Precise (clear and not vague statements directed toward goal accomplishment)
- Made to include a determined time frame (for example, one month, one year)
- Realistic (accomplishable within available time frame and resources)
- Sequenced (logical flow of steps is helpful in reaching the goal)

- Preferably written (writing out objectives enhances clarity and provides a documented record for future reference)
- Proactive (use of action verbs and self-driven)
- Measurable (changes need to be monitored in concrete terms)
- Behaviorally oriented (implying specific behavior changes that need to be accomplished)

Example of an objective:

"I will be able to identify one *irrational belief* responsible for causing my work-related anxiety, *within the next one week,* and achieve proficiency in practicing *progressive muscle relaxation* (PMR), as evinced by a feeling of relaxation by my body, after ten minutes of daily practice, performed after coming home from work."

This objective may appear to be slightly verbose, but we have attempted to explain most of the attributes within this example. While formulating objectives for ourselves, only we can be the best judge of the criteria that need inclusion and the criteria that can be excluded.

Deciding Targets

In order to achieve practical accomplishment of goals and objective, we need to perform a number of day-to-day activities. Identifying these day-to-day activities in advance is important in planning. This process is known as deciding targets. An example of a target would be "I will, at 6:00 P.M., after returning from work, perform progressive muscle relaxation."

Now, with the help of Worksheet 10.1, you can set your goals and establish your objectives. Worksheet 10.2 has been designed to prioritize your objectives. Worksheet 10.3 will help you to decide upon daily targets in order to accomplish prioritized objectives. You can use the format presented in Worksheet 10.3 for deciding daily targets for different objectives from either photocopies of the worksheet or a separate blank sheet of paper.

Thoughts for Reflection 10.1 will help you to ponder some ideas to keep in mind before setting goals and establishing objectives. Box 10.1 presents some Eastern thoughts on obtaining results.

Thoughts for Reflection 10.1
Points to Ponder

Goal setting and establishing objectives . . .

. . . are not wishful thinking or daydreaming.

. . . are positive, and proactive.

. . . are an individual activity that no one else can do for us.

. . . are not something to regret about the past or worry about for the future.

. . . are a powerful tool for success in life.

. . . are an act of discipline.

. . . are effective for reducing stress, managing change, and promoting health.

* * * * *

Box 10.1 Eastern Views on Obtaining Results

Most of our stress is due to expectations of obtaining results arising from our actions. We are not sure what results we will get, and this uncertainty is often a source of fear, anxiety, and other forms of stress. According to Eastern philosophy, the results are bound to follow any action. This is the basic law of nature: the law of cause and effect. The uncertain nature of results is also mandatory. According to this theory results are dependent on the following three aspects:

- *Effort:* No result can occur without an *effort* on our part. *Effort* is the first and foremost step toward obtaining results.
- *Direction:* If our *effort* lacks an appropriate direction, then we shall not be able to obtain the necessary results. Therefore, having a *direction* or focus is important to achieving success in our *effort.*
- *Unknown Factor:* Even after applying an *effort* in an appropriate *direction,* success sometimes does not come. Such failures are due to the unknown factor that is operating in the universal system of law. Religious-minded people refer to this as God; Scientists attribute it to probability and chance. Without being unduly concerned about the semantics, the basic fact remains that we need to acknowledge and accept this inherent phenomenon. We then need to strengthen our mind and not be perturbed if the results do not go our way.

The only aspects over which we have control are *effort* and *direction.* Having applied our *effort* and having done so in the right *direction,* we need to think no further. We need to develop an attitude of bearing whatever the results may be. If they are good, we need to be thankful to the "Unknown"; if they are not to our expectation, we need to think what went wrong, how we can rectify anything, if at all, and accept the result with fortitude and grace. If the result has been negative, we also need to rethink about changing our *effort* and *direction,* that is, the behavior, if it is faulty.

* * * * *

Worksheet 10.1
Determining Goals and Objectives

Seek out a quiet place and complete this worksheet. You need to write out an optimum number of goals and objectives, that is, not to have too few or too many. *It is also important to write these out.* You need to periodically reexamine, reassess, and redefine your goals and objectives. You could make photocopies of this basic format or work on a separate sheet of paper.

DAY AND DATE: ______________________________

A. Setting goals.

Personal goal:

____

____

____

Professional goal:

____

____

____

Social goal:

____

____

____

Spiritual goal:

____

____

____

Worksheet 10.1 Determining Goals and Objectives (cont'd)

B. Establishing objectives.

Objectives for personal goals:

Objectives for professional goals:

Worksheet 10.1 Determining Goals and Objectives (cont'd)

Objectives for social goals:

Objectives for spiritual goals:

* * * * *

Worksheet 10.2
Prioritizing Your Objectives

Now prioritize your objectives from all four categories in the space that follows:

	More Important	*Less Important*
More Changeable		
Less Changeable		

FEEDBACK ON WORKSHEET 10.2

Objectives relating to behavior changes that are more changeable and more important need to be our *first* priorities. Objectives that are more important and less changeable constitute our *second* priority. The *third* priority is objectives that are less important but more changeable. Less changeable and less important objectives need to be *ignored.*

* * * * *

Worksheet 10.3
Deciding Targets

Having prioritized your objectives, you now need to make a daily list of targets that will help you accomplish the objectives selected. Since this is a daily activity, you can practice on a blank sheet of paper or make photocopies of this worksheet for repeated use.

DAY AND DATE: ______________________________

Time	*Targets*

* * * * *

Finding the Best Techniques That Suit Your Goals

All of us are different entities in ourselves. Our personalities, our biological constitution, our behaviors, our values, our attitudes, and our beliefs are unique. Likewise, our goals are also bound to be unique and personal. There may be a similarity of pattern in our attributes and goals with other individuals, but ultimately this set of attributes that each one of us has is totally unique and specific in itself. Therefore, as we have already seen, it is important to identify stress management and reduction techniques that suit this uniqueness in each person's individuality and goals.

Worksheet 10.4 has been designed to provide you with an opportunity to identify and practice stress management and reduction techniques that suit your goals and "fit" your own unique individuality. These techniques, if practiced with *regularity* and *commitment,* are bound to produce beneficial results in achieving your goals in life.

Thoughts for Reflection 10.2 will help you reinforce a sense of commitment in order to keep up with the plan decided upon.

Thoughts for Reflection 10.2
Promise to Myself

Let me make a promise to myself, for my own good, that . . .

. . . I shall make an effort to practice what I have learned.

. . . I shall be disciplined and proactive in my approach.

. . . I shall remain optimistic and positive about life.

. . . I shall have faith in myself, my goals, and the techniques that I have learned.

. . . I shall be enthusiastic and implement my plans with zeal.

. . . I shall wear a cheerful countenance at all times and greet everyone around me with a smile.

. . . I shall bless everyone around me, even if they may appear to be my enemies.

. . . I shall devote all of my time to self-improvement—so much so that I will have no time to find mistakes in others.

. . . I shall have no unrealistic expectation from people and situations around me.

. . . I shall try to understand more often than to be understood.

. . . I shall be so strong that no worry over the future overpowers me and no past event disturbs my peace.

. . . I shall be relaxed, happy, and contented in my disposition with my present.

* * * * *

Worksheet 10.4
Stress Management and Reduction Techniques (SMART)
Practice Log

The SMART Practice Log has been designed to help learners experience and practice selected techniques. Record the information in the SMART Practice Log for at least one week or until you have gained sufficient practice with the desired techniques. The SMART Practice Log is an application tool.

What you need to do is to self-rate the techniques that you practice in terms of their *effectiveness, ease of application,* and *practical utility.* Rate these criteria on a scale of 1 to 5, that is, 1, very low; 2, low; 3, satisfactory; 4, high; and 5, very high. You may want to use the abbreviation for not applicable (NA) if you have not had enough opportunity to try the technique. Each technique has been provided with its respective worksheet number (WS No.), for ready reference.

Techniques	*Worksheet No.*	*Effectiveness*	*Ease of Application*	*Practical Utility*	*Reasons*
A. Relaxation techniques					
Yogic breathing or *Pranayama*	3.1				
Progressive muscle relaxation (PMR)	3.2				
Autogenic training	3.3				
Visual imagery	3.4				
B. Effective communication					
Communication assessment	4.1				
Situational communication	4.2				

Worksheet 10.4 Stress Management and Reduction Techniques (SMART) Practice Log (cont'd)

Techniques	*Worksheet No.*	*Effectiveness*	*Ease of Application*	*Practical Utility*	*Reasons*
Assessing assertive behavior	4.3				
Becoming assertive	4.4				
C. Anger management					
Assessment	5.1				
Managing your anger	5.2				
Learning active listening	5.3				
D. Coping with anxiety					
Assessment	6.1				
RET	6.2				
SKY	6.3				
Gestalt therapy	6.4				
Systematic desensitization	6.5				
E. Balanced diet and appropriate eating					
Awareness	7.1				
Plan	7.2				

Worksheet 10.4 Stress Management and Reduction Techniques (SMART) Practice Log (cont'd)

Techniques	*Worksheet No.*	*Effectiveness*	*Ease of Application*	*Practical Utility*	*Reasons*
F. Regular exercise					
Awareness	8.1, 8.2				
Exercise program	8.3				
G. Time management					
Awareness	9.1				
Practical steps	9.2				
H. Goals and objectives					
Determining	10.1				
Prioritizing	10.2				
Deciding targets	10.3				

FEEDBACK ON WORKSHEET 10.4

This worksheet has provided you with insight into determining techniques that best suit our individuality in terms of effectiveness, ease of applicability, and practical utility. You should also have discovered for yourself the reasons for some of the techniques not being successful for you. If these reasons are under your control, then you can work at modifying them. However, if these reasons are not under your control, you need to find out and practice other techniques that work. The key for success lies in consistency and determination in your efforts in regularly practicing these techniques. These techniques are more helpful in preventing and reducing stress than in managing stress. Therefore, the earlier the age for starting and incorporating these techniques into your life, the greater the resultant benefit.

* * * * *

Toward a Stress-Free Life

This workbook has provided you with techniques for preventing, reducing, and managing stress in your life. It is never too late to implement and practice these techniques regularly to obtain beneficial results. These results can be maximized if you incorporate these techniques within your daily life at a young age. Therefore, you should enter into an *agreement* with yourself to attain regularity in implementing the stress reduction plan in your life. If you attain this regularity for a continuous period of at least one year, it will become fully etched within your system. In order to achieve this continuity, you may reward yourself periodically with some tangible, self-decided rewards or incentives. Worksheet 10.5 has been designed to help you with this objective.

Another helpful way to ensure this regularity is through social networking or building social support. This social networking also contributes to managing your stress directly. You need to identify a close group of people around you who are available for listening empathically to your views and concerns, who can help to clarify questions you have, and who are willing to challenge you to grow if and when needed. Associating with such people helps to prevent, reduce, and manage stress in your life. Finally we would like to emphasize that by regularly practicing selected techniques identified through this workbook you can effectively manage your stress.

Worksheet 10.5
Self-Agreement

I, ____, hereby agree to practice selected techniques for stress management identified as beneficial and practical for me from the SMART Practice Log. I shall not procrastinate any further the implementation of these techniques in my life. I shall observe utmost regularity and a sense of discipline in implementing these techniques.

I shall periodically reward myself for this accomplishment. After attaining regularity for . . .

one month: I shall ____
(reward)

____

three months: I shall ____
(reward)

____

six months: I shall ____
(reward)

____

one year: I shall ____
(reward)

____

* * * * *

Stress Management Principle 10

Work on a plan; then the plan will work on you.

Summary Points

- Implementation of a plan is central for success.
- Self-motivation and degree of changeability are prerequisites for implementing a plan.
- The behaviors that are more important and more changeable deserve your first priority in implementation.
- You need to take stock of all your resources before you implement a plan. This process includes soliciting help from other people close to you and obtaining necessary material resources.
- Goals are an indication of what you want to accomplish in your life. They cover four different spheres of life, namely, personal, professional, social, and spiritual.
- Goal analysis or goal setting is a procedure useful in helping you describe the meaning of what you want to achieve in terms of attitude and understanding.
- Maslow's hierarchy of needs theory on motivation identifies five levels of needs: physiological, security, love, self-esteem, and self-actualization.
- Alderfer's ERG theory describes the core needs of existence, relatedness, and growth.
- Objectives can be defined as concerted, directed, focused, step-by-step efforts at achieving goals.
- Some attributes in establishing objectives include being precise, made to include a determined time frame, realistic, sequenced, proactive, preferably written, measurable, and behaviorally oriented.
- Deciding targets includes planning for the various day-to-day activities required in accomplishing goals and objectives.
- According to Eastern philosophy, success in any enterprise is dependent upon effort, direction, and an unknown factor.
- Regular practice of techniques described in this workbook will help you in preventing, reducing, and managing your stress.

References and Further Readings

Addington, J. E. (1977). *All about goals and how to achieve them.* Marina del Rey, CA: DeVorss.

Alderfer, C. (1969, May). An empirical test of a new theory of human needs. *Organizational Behavioral and Human Performance,* 142–175.

Green, L. G., & Kreuter, M. W. (1991). *Health promotion planning: An educational and environmental approach* (2nd ed.). Mountain View, CA: Mayfield.

Liebler, J. G., Levine, R. E., & Rothman, J. (1992). *Management principles for health professionals* (2nd ed.). Gaithersburg, MD: Aspen.

Mager, R. F. (1972). *Goal analysis.* Belmont, CA: Fearon Publishers/Lear Siegler.

Maslow, A. (1954). *Motivation and personality.* New York: Harper and Row.

Maslow, A. (1962). *Toward a psychology of being.* Monterey, CA: Brooks/Cole.

Robbins, S. P. (1989). *Organizational behavior: Concepts, controversies, and applications* (8th ed.). Englewood Cliffs, NJ: Prentice Hall.

LIST OF STRESS MANAGEMENT PRINCIPLES

1. **It is not the stressor but your perception of the stress that is important.**
2. **You need to become aware before considering change.**
3. **Make relaxation a part of your life.**
4. **Think first before passing judgment.**
5. **Balancing your anger balances your life.**
6. **Wipe out anxiety before it wipes you out.**
7. **Enjoy balanced meals at regular times and cherish the gift.**
8. **Start an exercise program and keep exercising regularly.**
9. **Do it now!**
10. **Work on a plan; then the plan will work on you.**

* * * * *

Guide to Pronunciation of Foreign Language Words

Abhnivesha, 21 əbh-nē′-vāsh
Adhi, 21, 33 ä′-dē
Adhibhotik, 21 ädhi-bhô-tik
Adhidevik, 21 ädhi-de-vik
Adhyatmik, 21 ädhyät′-mik
Agna Chakra, 75 ägna-chäk′-rä
Ahankara, 21, 33 əhn′-kärə
Ananda, 67 ä-nända
Asaana, 73 äsana
Asmita, 21 əs-mitä′
Asthangayoga, 73 ästhan-yoog
Atharva, 21 əth′-ərv
Atman, 21, 33 ätmə
Avidya, 21, 33 ä-vid′-yä
Ayurvedic, 21 ä-yoor-vā′-dəc
Bhagvad Gita, 21 bhəg-vəth′ gētä
Bhakti Yoga, 74 bhäktē-yoog
Brahma Sutras, 21 brəhm-so͞o′-tra
Chakra Yoga, 74 chäk′-rä yoog
Chakras, 73 chäk′-räs
Charaka Samhita, 21 chə-rəkə sə-nhitä′
Dharana, 73 dhər-ənə
Dhyana, 73 dhy-ənə
Dukha, 21, 33 doo-khə′
Dvesha, 21 dvāsh
Estresse, 11 es-tress-ē
Gyana, 22 gyä-nə
  Yoga, 74 yoog
Hatha Yoga, 74 hath-ä yoog
Kama, 21, 33 käm
Karma Yoga, 74 kər′-mə yoog
Kaya Kalpa, 75 kə-yä kal-pa
Klesa, 21, 33 klā-shə
Kriya Yoga, 74, 75, 103 krī-yä yoog
Kumbhaka, 76 kumb-haka
Kundalini Shakti, 73, 75
  kun-da-lēnē shə-ktē′
Manusmriti, 21 mån-o͞o-is-mrā-*thi*
Mooladhara, 75 mool-əd-hərə
Mudra Yoga, 74 mo͞o-drə yoog
Niyama, 73 nī-yäm
Prajanparadha, 21, 33 prə-jən-pərədə′
Pranayama, 73, 76, 79–81, 103
  pränä-yâm
Pratihara, 73 prät-i-hərə
Prosupta, 22 prō-so͞optə
Puraka, 76 pur-əkə′
Puranas, 21 poo-rän
Raga, 21 räg
Raja Yoga, 74 rəjə yoog
Rechaka, 76 rec-həkə
Relaxare, 71 re-lax-āre
Rig, 21 rigg
Rinzai Zen, 75 rin-zhäi′ zhən
Sadhana, 22 sä′-*th*nä
Sahasrara, 74, 75 səh-əs-rar
Sama, 21 säm
Samadhi, 73 sä-mädhi
  Bhavana, 22 bhəv-nə
Samkhya-yoga, 21 sän-khy yoog
Shanti Yoga, 75 shən-ti yoog
Soto Zen, 75 sō-tō′ zhən
Srimad Bhagvatam, 21
  shrē′-məd bhä-vətəm′
Stresse, 11 stress-ē
Strictus, 11 stric-tus
Susruta Samhita, 21 so͞osh-ro͞othä sə-nhitä′
Tantaras, 21 tənt′-ra
Tonu, 22 tô-no͞o
Trisna, 21, 33 trē-shnä′
Udara, 22 o͞o-dər
Upanishads, 21 upä-ni-shads
Veda(s), 21, 73 vā′-das
  Atharva, 21 əth′-ərv
  Rig, 21 rigg
  Sama, 21 säm
  Yajur, 21 yə′-jo͞or
Vichchinna, 22 vi-chinə
Vidya, 22 vid′-yä
Yajur, 21 yə′-jo͞or
Yama, 73 yäm
Yoga, 73–75, 103 yoog
  Asthanga, 73 ästhan
  Bhakti, 74 bhäktē
  Chakra, 74 chäk′-rä
  Gyana, 74 gyä-nə
  Hatha, 74 hath-ä
  Karma, 74 kər′-mə
  Kriya, 74, 75, 103 krī yä
  Mudra, 74 mo͞o-drə
  Raja, 74 rəjə
  Shanti, 75 shən-ti
Yogasutras, 21, 73 yoog-so͞o-trä
Zazen, 75 zä-zhən
Zen, 75 zhən
  Rinzai, 75 rin-zhäi′
  Soto, 75 sō-tō′
  Za, 75 zä

Pronunciation Key

Symbol	*Key Words*	*Symbol*	*Key Words*
a	asp, fat, parrot	b	bed, fable, dub, ebb
ā	ape, date, play, break, fail	d	dip, beadle, had, dodder
ä	ah, car, father, cot	f	fall, after, off, phone
		g	get, haggle, dog
e	elf, ten, berry	h	he, ahead, hotel
ē	even, meet, money, flea, grief	j	joy, agile, badge
		k	kill, tackle, bake, coat, quick
i	is, hit, mirror	l	let, yellow, ball
ī	ice, bite, high, sky	m	met, camel, trim, summer
		n	not, flannel, ton
ō	open, tone, go, boat	p	put, apple, tap
ô	all, horn, law, oar	r	red, port, dear, purr
oo	look, pull, moor, wolf	s	sell, castle, pass, nice
o͞o	ooze, tool, crew, rule	t	top, cattle, hat
yo͞o	use, cute, few	v	vat, hovel, have
yoo	cure, globule	w	will, always, sweat, quick
oi	oil, point, toy	y	yet, onion, yard
ou	out, crowd, plow	z	zebra, dazzle, haze, rise
u	up, cut, color, flood	ch	chin, catcher, arch, nature
ur	urn, fur, deter, irk	sh	she, cushion, dash, machine
		th	thin, nothing, truth
ə	a in ago	*th*	then, father, lathe
	e in agent	zh	azure, leisure, beige
	i in sanity	ŋ	ring, anger, drink
	o in comply	ʾ	[indicates that a following l
	u in focus		or n is a syllabic consonant,
ər	perhaps, murder		as in *cattle* (kat''l), *Latin* (lat''n)

Foreign Sounds

ȧ This symbol, representing the *a* in French *salle*, can best be described as intermediate between (a) and (ä).

ë This symbol represents the sound of the vowel cluster in French *coeur* and can be approximated by rounding the lips as for (ō) and pronouncing (e).

ö This symbol variously represents the sound of *eu* in French *feu* or of *ö* or *oe* in German *blöd* or *Goethe* and can be approximated by rounding the lips as for (ō) and pronouncing (ā).

ô̂ This symbol represents a range of sounds between (ô) and (u); it occurs typically in the sound of the *o* in French *tonne* or German *korrekt;* in Italian *poco* and Spanish *torero*, it is almost like English (ô), as in *horn.*

ü This symbol variously represents the sound of *u* in French *duc* and in German *grün* and can be approximated by rounding the lips as for (ō) and pronouncing (ē).

kh This symbol represents the voiceless velar or uvular fricative as in the *ch* of German *doch* or Scots English *loch.* It can be approximated by placing the tongue as for (k) but allowing the breath to escape in a stream, as in pronouncing (h).

H This symbol represents a sound similar to the preceding but formed by friction against the forward part of the palate, as in German *ich.* It can be made by placing the tongue as for English (sh) but with the tip pointing downward.

n This symbol indicates that the vowel sound immediately preceding it is nasalized; that is, the nasal passage is left open so that the breath passes through both the mouth and the nose in voicing the vowel, as in French *mon* (mōn). The letter *n* itself is not pronounced unless followed by a vowel.

r This symbol represents any of various sounds used in languages other than English for the consonant *r.* It may represent the tongue-point trill or uvular trill of the *r* in French *reste* or *sur,* German *Reuter,* Italian *ricotta,* Russian *gorod,* etc.

' The apostrophe is used after final *l* and *r,* in certain French pronunciations, to indicate that they are voiceless after an unvoiced consonant, as in *lettre* (let'r'). In Russian words the "soft sign" in the Cyrillic spelling is indicated by (y'). The sound can be approximated by pronouncing an unvoiced (y) directly after the consonant involved, as in *Sevastopol* (se' väs tô̂' pəl y').

* * * * *

Index